This book
is for you if you have been told by your doctor that you
have high blood pressure. It explains why you must
immediately take preventive steps even if you feel
perfectly all right. An elevated pressure may be a warning
signal of a serious cardiovascular disorder in its first stage
or an established chronic condition. If, and only if, high
blood pressure is detected and treated in time can serious
consequences like stroke, heart attack, and kidney failure
be prevented.

This volume in the *Medical Adviser Series* tells you how
you can find out whether you have high blood pressure,
what your doctor can do about it, and what you yourself
can do to bring it back to normal. Your doctor can help
you work out a treatment plan to bring the condition under
control. As a rule this plan will put you on regular
medication, seek to isolate and eliminate the factors in
your life that constitute a health hazard—your individual
risk factors—and, if indicated, propose changes in your
habits and your diet.

In its early stages high blood pressure is an asymptomatic disease,—i.e., a disease without overt symptoms,—yet
25% of all those who have it die as a result of it. However,
if you have high blood pressure and follow the advice
given here you will be able to lead a normal, productive
life.

Hanns Peter Wolff, M.D.
was born in Tsingta, China, in 1914. He studied medicine
in Breslau and Munich, Germany, and now is the director
of the 1st Department of Medicine of the University of
Mainz. He has lectured or held visiting professorships at
the universities of Dallas, Boston, Palo Alto, New York,
Rochester, and Minneapolis. He is a member of many
international medical societies, the co-founder and deputy
chairman of the German League for the Prevention of
High Blood Pressure, and chairman of the Scientific
Council of the German Federal Chamber of Medicine.

Speaking of:
High Blood Pressure

The
Medical
Adviser Series

Medical
Adviser
Series

Hanns P. Wolff, M.D.

Speaking of:
High
Blood
Pressure

A Comprehensive Guide for
Hypertensives and Their Partners

Translated by: Jean Steinberg

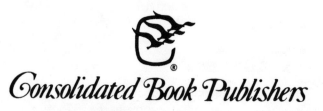

Consolidated Book Publishers

NEW YORK • CHICAGO

Library of Congress Catalog Card Number: 78-72873
ISBN: 0-8326-2235-4

Originally published in German under the title *Sprechstunde: Bluthochdruck,* copyright © 1978 by Gräfe und Unzer Verlag, München.

Contents

High Blood Pressure— the Silent Danger

More people die of high blood pressure than of cancer and tuberculosis combined

The devastating epidemics of the past—cholera, pestilence, bubonic plague, and tuberculosis—have disappeared almost entirely. They have been replaced by the no less frightening diseases of modern life. One of the most widespread of these is high blood pressure.

widespread disease

About 20% of all adults suffer from high blood pressure, and according to statistics the number keeps on growing. About 40% of all deaths below the age of 65 are due to the consequences of high blood pressure. And about 40% of all early retirements are due to cardiovascular diseases, of which high blood pressure is a frequent cause.

Were you aware of these facts and figures?

One out of every five persons has high blood pressure–but one-third of patients are not aware of it

11

Often un-
detected

The number of undetected cases of hypertension is still too high. Many people with high blood pressure are not familiar with the danger this presents to their life.

Why is high blood pressure dangerous?

Can result in
heart failure

The higher the blood pressure, the harder the heart has to work to keep on pumping against increasing resistance. If, in the course of time, the heart muscle tires, weakness and finally failure of the heart can result. Because of the enormous burden it puts on the arteries, high blood pressure adds to their wear and tear, especially in the target organs, the brain, coronary, and kidney vessels. Stroke and myocardial infarction (heart attack) therefore are frequent and dangerous consequences of untreated hypertension. A fatal stroke or heart attack is twice as great for people with untreated hypertension as for those with normal blood pressure of the same age.

Did you know how dangerous high blood pressure is?

How to recognize high blood pressure

Silent danger

High blood pressure is a "silent danger" because there are no typical symptoms sending out early warning signals. On the contrary: many people feel well and energetic despite their high blood pressure. There is only one way of finding out whether or not your blood pressure is normal and that is to have it checked. Blood pressure measurements must be repeated at least once a year. If an elevated pressure is detected in time, prompt treatment can help prevent the

12

possible fatal consequences.
What is your blood pressure?

How can the dangerous consequences of high blood pressure be prevented?

No heroic measures necessary

Bringing the blood pressure down relieves the strain on the heart and arteries; this lessens and often eliminates the dangerous consequences of elevated pressure. With proper treatment high blood pressure can be normalized, or at least brought down to a tolerable level. The treatment does not call for any heroic measures: regular checking of the blood pressure, a few generally painless changes in one's eating and living habits, taking the prescribed medication every day. If detected and treated in time, hypertension should not stop you from leading a normal and productive life. All that is required is determination and close doctor-patient cooperation.

Do you suffer from high blood pressure? If so, follow the treatment plan worked out by your doctor.

How can you protect yourself against high blood pressure?

Runs in the family

A genetic predisposition is a frequent cause of high blood pressure. It "runs in the family." If you have a family history of high blood pressure caution is advisable. The way you live can have a bearing on whether or when you will develop high blood pressure. If you are overweight you are a more likely candidate. Also, a high-sodium intake, psychological stress, agitation, and hyperactivity can exacerbate an existing tendency. Losing weight, cutting down on salt in the diet, and avoiding unnecessary

13

stress are useful precautions to help you keep your pressure down.

Do you have a tendency toward high blood pressure? If you do, change your way of life in time.

Why this book was written

I have written this book because I know that the chances of successful treatment are great in well-informed patients who understand the importance of close cooperation with their doctor.

Both the author and publisher have devoted much thought to the structure of this volume. Therefore, read the chapters in the order they have set up so as to gain a comprehensive understanding of all problems connected with high blood pressure.

1. Threats to Our Cardiovascular System

Cardiovascular Death

Modern hazards

Modern life offers many conveniences and comforts not dreamed of by our grandparents. But we have paid a price for all this in the form of increased hazards and risks. Probably the greatest dangers we face are the diseases of the cardiovascular system and their often fatal complications—heart attack and stroke. Hardly a day goes by that we don't read or hear about some public figure or acquaintance who has suffered a fatal heart attack or a stroke.

Although in the United States there has been a slow decline in the incidence rates over the past fifteen years, the death toll from heart attacks and strokes is still too high.

What do We Mean by ''Risk Factors''?

When you drive while under the influence of alcohol the risk of accident increases. This means that your elevated

15

blood alcohol level has become a risk factor. Another example: chronic tonsillitis in childhood may cause rheumatic heart disease, inflammation of the joints, or kidney disease. This makes infected tonsils a risk factor.

Risk factor defined   A risk factor thus is a potentially harmful condition that could trigger a specific disease or disability. People who have high risk factors are more likely to contract these diseases, and in a more serious form, than those who don't.

The high incidence of cardiovascular diseases has spurred an all-out search for their causes and the conditions that precipitate them. We know for a fact that more risk factors are found in people who have had heart attacks or strokes than in those who have not.

In recent years we have learned more and more about the nature of various risk factors and their effect on the cardiovascular system. Among them, harmful nutritional habits, specific metabolic disorders, blood vessel disease, and possibly emotional stress.

Risk factors

High blood pressure (hypertension)
Abnormal fat metabolism:
a. High serum cholesterol (hypercholesterolemia)
b. High serum triglyceride (hypertriglyceridemia)
Cigarette smoking
Diabetes
High serum uric acid level (hyperuricemia)
Overweight
Stress (possibly)

For more detailed information about the various risk factors and their relative importance, see pp. 24-26.

High Blood Pressure as a Risk Factor

The reason doctors and other concerned professionals stress the early detection and treatment of high blood pressure is its role in promoting arteriosclerotic disease.

Framingham study

It ranks first as a cause of stroke and heart attack and is a primary factor in congestive heart failure. This was established by the Framingham study. In a continuous study begun in 1949, the town of Framingham, Massachusetts, a suburb of Boston, was turned into a population laboratory to investigate the effects of various factors on the cardiovascular system of more than five thousand people. It was found that in the same age group the risk of congestive heart failure was six times greater for hypertensives than for persons whose blood pressure was normal. That explains why in the past, before we were able to treat high blood pressure effectively, almost 50% of all persons with high blood pressure died of congestive heart failure. Today myocardial infarction is the cause of death of about 30% of people suffering from high blood pressure, and about the same number have fatal strokes.

As the blood pressure goes up so does the threat to health. And if other risk factors are also present, the danger to heart and circulation increases proportionately. Thus a diabetic with high blood pressure is ten times more likely to suffer a heart attack than a diabetic with normal blood pressure.

San Francisco study

In a study conducted among a group of San Francisco longshoremen it was found that high blood pressure plus cigarette smoking was a particularly dangerous combination. The incidence of heart attacks was ten times greater among smokers with high blood pressure than among smokers whose blood pressure was normal. And we know that even with normal blood pressure the incidence of heart attacks is twice as high among smokers as among nonsmokers.

High blood pressure beyond any doubt is one of the most common and most dangerous diseases of modern life. And although we lack exact statistics about its incidence

17

and the number of undetected cases, we can safely assume that almost 15% of all adults in advanced countries, and about 20-25% of all persons above the age of forty, have high blood pressure. In other words, one out of every five adults who sees a doctor for any reason whatsoever is found to have high blood pressure. Above and beyond this alarming figure lies the equally disturbing number of undetected cases. Here we can only guess, but on the basis of what we know we can assume that as many as 30% of all cases of high blood pressure go undetected.

No warning signals

If this figure comes as a surprise to you then you should ask yourself whether you yourself are not perhaps one of those unknown cases. High blood pressure, an asymptomatic ailment, can continue over many years without sending out any typical warning signals. Usually its existence is discovered by accident, in the course of a visit to a doctor's office for some other reason. Strangely enough some doctors do not bother to take the blood pressure as a matter of course. In view of the many undetected cases, by sure to ask to have your blood pressure checked every time you see your doctor.

Other Risk Factors

The subject of this book is the risk of high blood pressure, which is itself a dangerous disease. If we also go into other risk factors in some detail, we do so because a risk factor generally does not exist all by itself, and because common sense dictates that we try to identify and eliminate all existing risk factors and potential hazards. To attack only one factor is as pointless as equipping your car with the very best safety belts money can buy while driving with worn tires and defective brakes.

We know that risk factors are closely linked to the way we live. High blood pressure, diabetes, and metabolic disorders are diseases of the prosperous society. Because

18

the malnourished peoples of the developing countries are generally too poor to "afford" these risk factors, cardiovascular diseases are not very common among them. But as their economic situation improves and they acquire some of the living standards of the industrial nations, their rate of cardiovascular disease also goes up.

Overeating causes over-weight

Excess weight. This promotes the development of various risk factors and thus, by itself, constitutes a serious health hazard. 85% of all diabetics, 80% of all persons with abnormal blood levels of cholesterol and/or triglycerides, 70% of all cases of hyperuricemia (an excess of uric acid in the blood), and 60% of all hypertensives are overweight. The major cause of overweight is overeating. A further cause is lack of exercise, the occupational disorder of so many who spend their working life behind desks, factory benches, or the wheel of a car.

To find out whether and how much you are overweight see the section on your risk profile, p. 26. For tips on reducing see p. 100.

Cholesterol and arterio-sclerosis

Abnormal fat metabolism. The serum fats, also known as lipids, supply the body with energy and building material. In part they are taken in with the food we eat and in part they are composed by the body itself. If, as a result of a poor diet, the body receives more fats than it needs, then the blood fat level rises.

A chronically high blood fat condition (hyperlipidemia) can trigger and accelerate the degenerative processes of the arterial wall—the condition we call arteriosclerosis. Two types of blood fats—cholesterol and triglycerides, and particularly cholesterol—play a crucial role in this. Cholesterol is largely produced by the body itself, but the blood cholesterol level is linked to our diet, to the type of fats we eat and the cholesterol contained in our food. The body is able to convert carbohydrates like sugar, flour, bread and bread products into fats known as triglycerides. Two Norwegian epidemiologists, Westlund and

19

Nicolaysen, found that middle-aged men with a blood cholesterol level of more than 250mg% run a higher than average risk of heart attack, and the risk increases substantially as the level rises. The cholesterol level has been called a *warning signal of unique predictive ability*.

A unique warning signal

Because an elevated blood triglyceride level may also be a hazard it should not be ignored.

Smoking. Cigarettes are a significant risk factor in cardiovascular disease according to a study of the World Health Organization made in 1965. And the Framingham study lends support to this finding. Whereas people who smoke one pack of cigarettes a day are three times as likely to suffer a heart attack than nonsmokers, the risk increases as consumption goes up; with chain smokers the chances for heart attacks are six times those of nonsmokers.

Hope for smokers

The most important information for the ex-smoker is the fact that the risk of heart attacks, within a short period of time, returns to the level of nonsmokers.

Diabetes. The Framingham study also makes clear that one out of every two diabetics sooner or later suffers blood vessel damage and runs an increased risk of heart attack. The incidence of hypertension among diabetics is greater than among non-diabetics in the same age group, and it is just as high for men with diabetes as for women. The link between the two risk factors, diabetes and hypertension, explains the relative frequency of coronary disease among people with both conditions. And there is a still more important association between untreated or inadequately treated diabetes and blood vessel disease (arteriosclerosis) of the legs; in extreme cases it can lead to diabetic gangrene and must be treated by amputation of toes or of the entire leg.

Hyperuricemia (the accumulation of uric acid in the blood). Hyperuricemia is a metabolic disorder with potentially

20

very painful consequences. The body converts this excess uric acid into tiny crystals which may lodge in the joint tissues. The result is the painful disease known as gout. As early as 1899 a French physician by the name of Huchard stated that this excess of uric acid affected not only the joints but also the arteries. Because hyperuricemia often appears associated with overweight as well as with high blood pressure, diabetes and abnormal fat metabolism, we are still not certain whether it deserves to be treated as a risk factor by itself. One important aspect is that people with high blood pressure are three times as likely to suffer coronary heart disease as hypertensives with normal uric acid levels in the blood.

A catch-all term

Stress. Stress has become a popular term used to explain everything from simple headaches to serious disorders. We hear and read about it at the dinner table and on TV talk shows, in the papers and magazines. But what does it mean? Professor H. Selye, the inventor of the stress concept, applied it to the protective "alarm mechanism" of the body against overburdening. Under stress the nervous system goes into "high gear" and triggers the production of large amounts of hormones to raise the body's defenses and resistance. Stress reactions can be set off by a vast array of different conditions—by cold and heat, infection and injuries, by psychological and emotional strain.

Whether this ordinary stress will turn into a permanent condition, i.e., into a constant stimulant of the defense mechanism, and whether this persistent pressure to operate at "high gear" will ultimately put an undue burden on the cardiovascular system depends on a variety of factors, primarily on the nature of the stress and on its impact and duration. Professor L. Levy of Sweden has compiled a list of the stresses of everyday life as defined by medical psychology. Among them are:

List of stresses

• The oppressive demands created by the conflicts about our "role" in our various life situations—i.e., our work, marriage, relationship with our parents, etc.

21

• The oppressive demands created by unanticipated and sudden changes in our lives, such as job changes and transfers, job insecurity, and similar radical inroads calling for major readjustments.

• The inability to adjust to new life situations and settings because of discrepancy between expectations and reality in business and personal life.

The stress-prone individual

Whether this sort of stress turns into a risk factor seems to depend on the individual, on his or her "stressability." Dr. M. Friedman and Dr. R. H. Rosenman have written a book in which they characterize the stress-prone individual as one who lives by the clock, who speaks rapidly and in a tense manner, who doesn't listen, who tries to do more than one thing at a time, who always wants to outdo others, who is unable to enjoy himself, who grinds his teeth. A person of this type lives rather dangerously; not so much the stress, but his own personality may constitute a risk factor.

Many readers will recognize themselves or others in this description. Yet much of this is merely a theory, a working hypothesis. Research on stress is still in its infancy, and the lack of objective research methods complicates matters. This is because stress, unlike other risk factors or blood pressure, cannot be measured in numbers, nor, unlike smoking does it lend itself to comparative studies. Just as some people are more thin-skinned than others, some are more prone to stress than others. In other words, different types of stress affect different people differently and evoke different physical reactions.

No conclusive proof

That is why medical science, although admitting that stress may be harmful, does not, in the absence of conclusive proof, accept it as the major causal factor of cardiovascular disease. Contrary to popular belief, stress plays a much smaller role as a risk factor than do poor dietary habits.

Professor Selye, in his book on stress, maintains that stress is not merely nervous tension. "The absence of stress is death," he writes, and goes on to say that it

22

matters little whether a given situation was triggered by pleasant or unpleasant circumstances; what matters rather is the adjustment required. As a physician in daily contact with people who have had to cope with highly stressful situations, he has been in a position to observe the effects on their health.

The widespread preoccupation with and misconceptions about stress as a risk factor have been further helped by the superficial coverage of the various media. It is for this reason that I have gone into this matter in some detail. I will return to it in the discussion on the causes of high blood pressure.

The Adverse Effects of Risk Factors

Arterio-
sclerosis

The relationship between risk factors and the cardiovascular system has been thoroughly studied. We know that they increase the development of arteriosclerosis, the underlying condition in most cardiovascular diseases. Arteriosclerosis, or hardening of the arteries, as it is commonly called, is the result of the strains and damages sustained by the walls of the arteries in the course of a lifetime. The crucial factor here is when they first appear and the extent of the damage. This is what determines our "biological" age as opposed to our chronological age, and on it depends what we are able to do, how old we look, and how well we feel.

Risk factors can accelerate and intensify the progression of arteriosclerosis. The elasticity and muscular structure of the arterial walls deteriorate and are replaced by scar tissue; lipid and calcium salt deposits enter (from the blood stream) the arterial wall. Blood clots begin to form along the interior walls; formerly elastic arteries turn into inflexible constricted tubes with thickened walls that interfere with the regular flow of oxygen and nutrients to target organs. As a result, the undernourished tissue cells

23

of the heart muscle deteriorate and die. The outcome of this process is the impaired functioning of the myocardium, and ultimately its failure. The three organs most endangered by these complications are—the heart, brain, and kidneys.

What About Your Risk Factors?

North American Pooling Project

The existence and prevalence of risk factors are fairly recent discoveries. Pioneering studies, particularly the one in Framingham, have contributed greatly to our awareness of them. In the course of the North American Pooling Project (which pooled data from the Framingham Study, the Albany, Tecumsah, Los Angeles, and Minneapolis Studies as well as those from the Chicago Gas Company and the Chicago Western Electric Company) 7,342 men between the ages of thirty and fifty-nine with no apparent health problems were examined. Of these, only 1,249 or 17% were found to be without two of the major risk factors of high blood pressure—cigarette smoking and hypercholesteremia. 45% of the men had at least one risk factor, 30% had two, and 8% had three.

All of us know people with at least one of these risk factors, for example, overweight diabetics who smoke or chain smokers who have high blood pressure. Perhaps you yourself are part of this high-risk group without knowing it. It is in your own best interest to find out whether you are or not. The questionnaire on p. 26, drawn up by Professor S. Heyden, a well-known epidemiologist, can help you find out. Not all of the factors on this questionnaire carry equal weight or are equally hazardous. Talk to your doctor about the significance of the various factors as they affect your health and your life.

We do not want to cause anxiety by our discussion of these risk factors, although we are aware that objective statements about health hazards are bound to create concern. Our purpose in calling your attention to this is to appeal to your common sense, to get you to act, to have regular physical checkups. Try to close the gap between awareness and action, what psychologists call cognitive dissonance: you know only too well the hazards of certain of your habits, yet you close your eyes to them and do nothing to change them.

Checklist for Risk Factors: Normal and High Levels

Cigarette smoker	Nonsmoker		
Height	Weight	Normal weight: Ideal weight:	
Systolic blood pressure (mm Hg)	Diastolic blood pressure (mm Hg)	Normal: Borderline: High pressure:	100-139 mm Hg systol. and 60-89 mm Hg diastol. 140-159mm Hg systol. and 90-94 mm Hg diastol. 160 mm Hg and above systolic or 95 mm Hg and above diastolic
Blood sugar (in mg%)		To age 49: Normal: Age 50 and up: Normal:	up to 100 mg% (fasting) or up to 110 mg% (not fasting) up to 110% (fasting) or up to 129 mg% (not fasting)
Fat level Cholesterol (in mg%) Triglyceride (mg%) fasting		Normal: Borderline: In need of treatment: Normal: Borderline: In need of Treatment:	up to 220 mg% 221-259 mg% from 260 mg% up to 150 mg% 150-180 mg% from 181 mg%
Uric acid (in mg%)	Men Women	Normal: Borderline: In need of treatment: Normal: Borderline: In need of treatment:	up to 6 mg% 6,1 mg%—7,0 mg% from 7,1 mg% up to 5,5 mg% 5,6 mg%—6,0 mg% from 6,1 mg%

These levels are important! Have your doctor check them and discuss the results with him!

2. Blood Pressure and the Cardiovascular System

How does cardio-vascular system work?

This book talks a lot about the blood circulation, the heart, and the arteries—and of course about blood pressure. You are undoubtedly familiar with all these terms. But do you know how the cardiovascular system functions, what it is supposed to do, and what role blood pressure plays in it?

In this chapter we will examine the structure and function of the cardiovascular system insofar as it relates to the causes and effects of high blood pressure and its treatment.

The Organism Blood Circulation Serves

To help you understand the function and operation of the cardiovascular system, the system directly affected by our blood pressure, let us compare it to a complicated, largely automated industrial plant with numerous highly specialized departments working together in close harmony. Some of these plant components, such as the motor system with its muscles and bones, perform specific, obvious functions. Others, like the lungs, intestines, and

27

kidneys, supply the necessary energy and eliminate waste products. To work smoothly, a plant composed of so many specialized departments needs an information and control center. This job is performed by a central computer-like organ, the brain, which is connected to the other organs by three networks of nerves which together form the central nervous system: the sensory nervous system, which regulates the sensory organs, the autonomic nervous system, which regulates the internal organs, and the peripheral nervous system, which is connected to the muscles and skin. These networks feed the brain a constant stream of information which the brain in turn evaluates and on the basis of which it sends out detailed operating instructions. This activity is only partly subject to voluntary decisions. A constant demand for voluntary decisions would put far too great a strain on the autonomic nervous system, which coordinates vital functions like breathing, circulation, digestion, and metabolism with the constantly changing needs of the entire organism. The actions of the autonomic nervous system are therefore largely involuntary, hence its name. Because one of its functions is the regulation of the blood pressure we will go into it in more detail at a later point.

The central nervous system

The Structure and Function of the Cardiovascular System

The complicated structure of our body requires an extensive supply network to assure the prompt and adequate delivery of vital supplies and the elimination of waste products.

The circula-tory system

The agency that furnishes this vital service is the circulatory system. It is made up of a branched-out network of "pipes" to which the tissue cells are attached. The fluid that flows through these "pipes," our blood, is

28

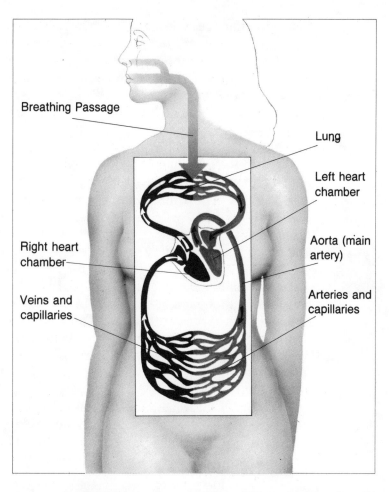

Breathing Passage

Lung

Left heart chamber

Right heart chamber

Aorta (main artery)

Veins and capillaries

Arteries and capillaries

Cardiovascular system. The heart consists of two independent chambers or ventricles and their atria. The right chamber pushes the blood into the lung vessels where it loads up with oxygen. The left chamber pumps the blood into the circulatory system, whose arteries and capillaries (here shown in simplified form) supply the body with blood.

composed of a protein-rich substance called blood plasma (60%) and of red blood cells called erthrocytes (40%). The blood plasma in liquid form carries all the nutrients, building and other materials required by the cells: sugar, fats, minerals, vitamins, and hormones. The red blood cells can be compared to minute cannisters containing red coloring (hemoglobin) that serves as a conduit of oxygen and carbon dioxide. The red blood cells carry the oxygen inhaled by the lungs to the cells of the organs and muscles. Without oxygen the cells cannot live and do their work. The metabolic system needs it to convert the food products (sugar, carbohydrates, fats) into energy. At the same time the cells must get rid of carbon dioxide, the metabolic waste, otherwise they would drown in it.

Red blood cells

The blood is kept in motion by a pump, the heart. A system of "pipes," originating from the heart, the arteries, transports the blood to the tissues; from there they branch out into a network of tiny vessels, the so-called capillaries. The blood of the capillaries bathes the cells, and they extract from it the supplies they need. In exchange, the cells deposit the metabolic wastes they had stored in the blood, which carries them away. The system of "pipes" that carry the waste materials are called veins. In the course of its passage the blood goes through organs that detoxify the wastes (the liver) and take care of their excretion (the kidneys).

In order for this ingenious transportation system to function, the individual components must perform a variety of complex operations. That explains the differences in their structure.

The Arteries

Carry blood to all cells

The arteries play a crucial role in the origin of high blood pressure and its dangerous consequences. Not only do the arteries have to carry the blood from the heart to all organs, but they play a further vital role in the regulation, distribution, and pressure of the blood flow. The burden of this function falls on the arterial walls. There are two basic types of arteries:

Types of arteries

- *elastic* and
- *muscular.*

The elastic arteries are so named because their walls are composed of a vast number of elastic fibers. This enables them to function like a compressed air tank and distributor. The rhythmic pumping of the heart sends out the blood in regular intervals rather than in an even flow. The elastic arteries, particularly the largest artery—the aorta—transform this pulsating jet stream into a smooth, continuous flow. This guarantees an even blood supply to the target organs and muscles. Because of the elasticity of their walls, these arteries work like the bellows of a bagpipe. On the one side air is pumped in rhythmically and then, when pressure is applied to the air bag, it flows out evenly on the other side.

At the periphery of the arterial circulatory system the elastic arteries turn into muscular arteries, which, in addition to circulating the blood, must also see to its distribution. The powerful muscles in their walls enable them to expand (dilate) or contract and in this way to increase or decrease the flow of blood to specific parts of the body as needed. The expansion (dilatation) or contraction of the artery naturally affects the resistance of the arterial wall. The combined resistance of all the peripheral muscular arteries is called peripheral arterial resistance, a significant factor in the level of blood pressure in the arterial system. We will hear more about this resistance in our discussion of the causes and treatment of high blood pressure.

Peripheral arterial re-sistance

The smallest muscular arteries are called arterioles. They branch out into a network of still more minute vessels, the capillaries, which bring nutrients to the cells and carry off waste materials.

The Veins

The venous capillaries—that portion of the capillary system leading away from the tissues—unite with the large thin-walled blood vessels known as veins. The flow of blood in the capillary network is very deliberate; the venous blood returning to the heart moves at a very slow pace, almost without any pressure. The veins merge into two major trunks, the *venae cavae*. The superior *vena cava* returns the blood from the head, neck, and arms to the heart, and the inferior *vena cava* returns the blood from the trunk and legs; both these veins lead into the right atrium of the heart.

Blood returns to heart

The Heart

The heart is a muscle approximately the size of a man's closed fist located within the chest cavity just left of center between the lungs. It is divided into two equal cavities separated by a wall of muscle: the "left" heart and the "right" heart; each half in turn is divided into two chambers: the upper one is called the atrium and a lower portion is known as the ventricle. A system of valves separates the atrias and ventricles and regulates the flow of blood into and out of the heart.

A coupled double pump

The structure of the heart can best be compared to a coupled double pump. As a matter of fact the left and right heart are two mechanically independent pumping stations that form a single organ. And like the heart, the circulatory system is also made up of two separate parts: pulmonary circulation serving the lungs, and the systemic circulation serving the body as a whole. The right heart pumps blood into the pulmonary circulation and the left heart supplies the systemic circulation (see illustration p. 33). The division serves a vital function: the "exchange of gases" between air, blood, and tissues. As was previously mentioned, the body cells must be supplied with oxygen

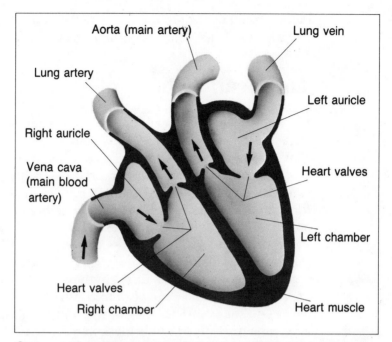

Labels on the diagram:
- Aorta (main artery)
- Lung vein
- Lung artery
- Left auricle
- Right auricle
- Heart valves
- Vena cava (main blood artery)
- Left chamber
- Heart valves
- Heart muscle
- Right chamber

Cross-section of the heart and direction of blood flow. The deoxygenated blood returns through the venous system and the *vena cava* to the heart via the right atrium. It reaches the right ventricle through the tricuspid valve, from where it is pumped into the pulmonary artery and its branches. The oxygenated blood from the lungs reaches the left atrium via the pulmonary vein and from there, via the mitral valve, flows into the left ventricle. From there it is pumped into the aorta and its branches. A system of valves separates the right ventricle from the pulmonary artery and the left ventrical from the aorta.

Exchange of oxygen and carbon dioxide

and be allowed to rid themselves of carbon dioxide in order to live. The supply and excretion of these two gases takes place in the following fashion. The right ventricle receives the deoxygenated blood from the *vena cava* and pumps it into the pulmonary circulation. The extensive capillary network promotes the rapid exchange between the air cells (alveoli) in the lungs and the deoxygenated blood pumped in by the heart; the red blood cells eliminate the carbon dioxide and take up oxygen. The oxygenated blood is then carried to the heart by the pulmonary vein, and then the heart sends it out into the blood stream.

The Heart Action

Atria and ventricles work in harmony

If this exchange of gases is to function smoothly, the two atria and the two ventricles must work in close harmony. This harmony is achieved by the coordinated action of the atria and ventricles: the two atria release their blood simultaneously into the adjacent ventricles, and these in turn simultaneously pump the blood into both the pulmonary and systemic arteries. The system controlling this coordinated action operates like an electrical generator and distributor. The generator, located in the region of the atria, sends forth rhythmical electrical impulses which cause the atria to contract and release the blood into the ventricles. Then, with only a minimum delay, the distributor sends these impulses to the blood-filled ventricles, whereupon they release the blood into the circulation. This electrical "conduction system" is the most sensitive part of the heart pump. That is why irregular heart beat—arrhythmia—is often the first indication of a possible circulatory disturbance or a malfunctioning heart muscle.

Tremendous work

In order to gain an idea of the tremendous work done by the heart let us try to visualize its operation. The volume of blood released by the ventricles with each thrust of the pump—the heart beat—is a measurable quantity. The heart-beat frequency, the number of heart beats per minute, normally ranges between 60 and 80. Under conditions of stress or physical exertion this rate can double. One measure of the work performed by the heart is the per minute volume, i.e., the amount of blood pumped out per minute. While resting, this volume ranges between 3 and 5 quarts, an amount large enough to fill an 80 by 165 foot pool in about one year, and can increase from 3 to 5 times this amount with physical work or

34

exercise depending on the individual condition.

0.1 horse-power pump

The heart is a pump with the strength of 0.1 horse-power. It does not only perform strenuous labor but, unlike other muscles, it must do so throughout life. This makes it utterly dependent on a constant adequate supply of oxygen and necessary fuels. The job of assuring this flow falls to the coronary arteries surrounding the heart. They branch out from the aorta, immediately behind the exit from the left heart, into the muscles of both the left and the right heart. As mentioned earlier, the coronary vessel system is a danger zone for people with risk factors—particularly for those with high blood pressure.

Blood Pressure and Its Functions

The purpose of blood pressure

What is the purpose of blood pressure? Obviously, the heart and circulation are assigned the job of supplying all organs of the body with blood. They can do this job only if the basic material—i.e., blood, is available and then, if there is enough pressure to send it on its way. Since the available amount of blood is constant—about 4-5 quarts in adults—the pressure must be able to adjust to the changing requirements of the body. This means it must not fall below a certain minimum level—a condition that can lead to hypotension with its concomitant problems—and that it must be able to react promptly to sudden demands. The cardiovascular system has two simple mechanisms to help it adjust to fluctuating demands for blood by target organs: one is by decreasing or increasing the amount of blood pumped into the circulation, the per minute volume, and the other is by decreasing or increasing the resistance of the muscular arteries through contraction or dilation. This seemingly simple regulatory mechanism is coordinated by a complex control system, which perhaps can best be understood if we first look at the behavior pattern of blood pressure in different everyday situations.

35

When Does Blood Pressure Go Up, and When Does It Go Down?

Pressure never constant

If you are worried about your blood pressure reading, remember this: blood pressure is never constant; it is a condition that changes according to the needs and requirements of the body, and it does so frequently in the course of every day. Whether it goes up or down depends on a wide variety of different factors.

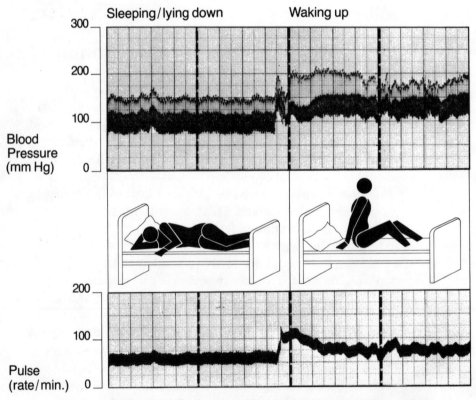

Increase in blood pressure upon awakening. Tonus of the sympathetic nervous system is heightened, resulting in a temporary increase in blood pressure and pulse rate.

The lowest pressure readings normally occur while sleeping. During the day with its physical and psychological demands and strains, pressure usually goes up, adjusting constantly to different requirements and muscle *Pressure* activities. Let us take two examples:

while When we stand erect, the blood, because of its weight, *standing* flows down to the lower extremities. At the same time, the

| | Eating | Bowel Movement | Resting | Sleeping |

Blood Pressure (mm Hg): 275, 200, 100, 0

Pulse (rate/min.): 200, 100, 0

Changes in blood pressure in various everyday situations. The two illustrations show how blood pressure adjusts to the different needs of the organism. Blood pressure is lowest during sleep, higher during physical activity and psychic stress.

blood pressure goes down and could continue to do so to the point of danger if the regulatory mechanism of our circulation would not automatically raise the pressure and maintain it at a normal level by constricting the peripheral arteries. If this mechanism works too slowly or not satisfactorily it can cause a temporary blood shortage in the brain. The result is a feeling of light-headedness and dizziness. Most of us have at one time or another

37

experienced this harmless sensation after getting up suddenly or after having stood for a long time.

Pressure while climbing stairs

In a similar manner the circulation adjusts to physical activity. If, for example, you climb a flight of stairs the demand for oxygen and, therefore, for blood by the leg muscles increases. To meet this demand your heart begins to pump more rapidly; at the same time your peripheral

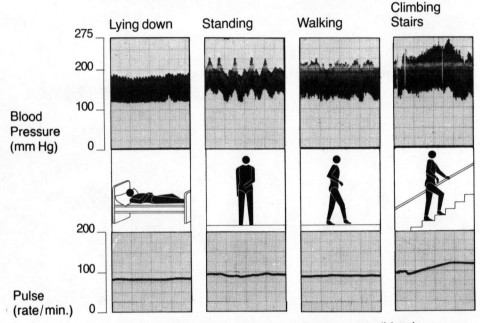

Drawings based on monitored endurance tests (blood pressure telemetry) conducted by Dr. Kroenig, one of the author's former co-workers at the Medical Clinic and Polyclinic in Maine.

arteries constrict, with the exception of the vessels of the legs, which dilate. Your blood pressure goes up and the blood flow to your legs increases. Once you have reached the top and rest, the blood requirements of your leg muscles return to normal, and with it the heart activity and blood pressure.

We know from experience how excitement can affect circulation: "pounding heartbeats", accompanied by a definite increase in blood pressure. That holds true

38

regardless of the cause, whether pleasure or pain, shame or fear, or simple irritation over being caught in a traffic jam when you're in a hurry or feel pressured on your job. This rise in blood pressure under conditions of psychological stress or nervous tension helps you to keep under control in critical situations by making you more alert and responsive. When the specific cause of the excitement is removed or comes to an end, the blood pressure returns to its baseline level.

How the Blood Pressure Is Regulated

How does the organism solve the problem of adjusting the pressure and distribution of arterial blood to the constantly changing demands of its organs? In regulating blood pressure nature resorts to a principle of modern technology—and most likely has done so for millions of years—known as "regulator with feedback."

The walls of the large arteries, particularly the aorta and the kidney arteries, are lined with pressure-sensitive cells, something like tiny gauges. These "pressure receptors," to give them their scientific name, are connected by nerve channels with the circulation center of the brain, to which they transmit information about the pressure relationships in the different sectors of the arterial system. The circulation collates these with other vital data and reports it receives, such as metabolic information from the blood and brain impulses. The circulation center is linked to the muscular arteries and heart by the "sympathetic" channels of the autonomic nervous system. If an increase in blood pressure is necessary, the center sends appropriate signals to the bulblike terminals of the sympathetic nerve fibers in the target organs. The nerve fibers act somewhat like specialized laboratories with enormous production and storage capacity, and immediately release quantities of noradrenalin. This is a hormone that

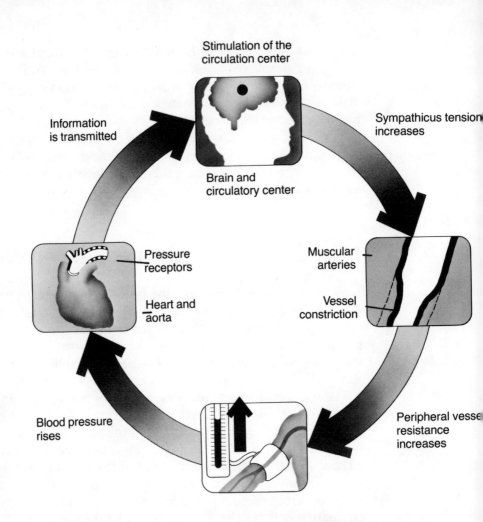

Stimulation of the
circulation center

Sympathicus tension
increases

Information
is transmitted

Brain and
circulatory center

Muscular
arteries

Pressure
receptors

Vessel
constriction

Heart and
aorta

Blood pressure
rises

Peripheral vessel
resistance
increases

Regulation of blood pressure, showing feedback. Shows how
the organism solves the problem of adjusting the pressure and
distribution of arterial blood to the constantly changing blood supply
needs.

constricts the peripheral arteries and stimulates heart
activitiy. The hormone thus augments arterial resistance to
the flow of blood and the heart per minute volume. The
result is a rise in blood pressure. If the brain center data

analysis indicates that the reported blood pressure exceeds the demand, the signals abate, that is, the stimulation of the sympathetic channels diminishes and with it the noradrenalin production. To sum up, the controlling mechanism of blood pressure works as follows.

The circulation center is stimulated—sympathetic activity increases—vessels constrict—blood pressure increases—pressure receptors are stimulated— information goes to the circulation center—reversal— sympathetic activity decreases—blood vessels dilate— blood pressure decreases.

This closes the circle. If the system is activated by a sudden decrease in blood pressure, the cycle is reversed.

The functional unit of sympathetic nerve fibers and their noradrenalin-producing terminals in the heart and arterial walls are called the sympathetic-adrenergic system. This will be referred to repeatedly in the subsequent chapters because it plays a crucial role in the development of high blood pressure as well as in its treatment.

Systolic and Diastolic Pressure

Each time the blood pressure is checked, two figures are recorded: the upper, or systolic pressure, and the lower, or diastolic reading.

The heart in its rhythmic contractions sends out a stream of blood (pulse wave) to the peripheral arteries, where it can be felt as a "pulse." Depending on whether the heart contracts or dilates, the pressure in the arteries will be either higher or lower. Thus the pulse wave, like all waves, crests and then recedes. The highest value, caused

by the contraction (systole) of the heart chambers (ventricles) is called systolic pressure, and the lower corresponding to their dilation (diastole) is known as the diastolic pressure. (More about the method of measuring blood pressure will be found on p.108) Because the

41

respective levels of these two pressures, as well as their relationship to each other, furnish valuable clues to the physician both pressures are always taken. Blood pressure, like barometric pressure, is expressed in millimeters of mercury (mm Hg). A measurement of 130/85 mm Hg means a systolic pressure of 130 and a diastolic pressure of 85.

When Is Blood Pressure in the Normal Range and When Is It Elevated?

For a variety of reasons medical science has had difficulties in establishing a standard norm. First of all, there is the natural daily fluctuation mentioned earlier. The blood pressure of a normal person at rest can range from 95/65 mm Hg at night to 135/80 in the morning to 150/90 in the evening. Moreover, the blood pressure of many, though by no means all, people goes up with age but they do not suffer from hypertension. Also, blood pressure levels like other biological norms can be established only after taking the measurements many times in healthy individuals. But since the pressure levels of such persons vary enormously it is difficult to establish a rigid dividing line between normal (normotension) and high blood pressure (hypertension).

On the other hand, it is vital to establish firm upper normal limits, for without them we cannot detect high blood pressure nor evaluate the effectiveness of treatment. After much debate one has arrived at a rule of thumb to determine a valid norm:

*Rule of
thumb*

To determine the acceptable upper norm of systolic pressure
    age plus 100 (maximum 160 mm Hg)
To determine the acceptable upper norm of diastolic pressure
    90 mm Hg, regardless of age.

42

Thus, if you are forty years of age, your blood pressure should not exceed 140/90. If it is between 140/90 and 160/90, you should have your pressure checked every three to six months to make sure that there is no upward trend. A reading of 160/95 would certainly seem to indicate that you have high blood pressure.

Moderate divergences not unusual

Moderate divergences from the systolic standard values—from 20 to 30 mm Hg lower, and, if sixty years and older, of 10 to 20 mm Hg higher are not unusual and compatible with good health. (For more information about taking your blood pressure see p. 108.)

3. The Causes of High Blood Pressure

Elevated Blood Pressure Is Not Necessarily a Sign of Disease

Blood pressure not a constant factor

Before discussing the potential implications of an elevated blood pressure it is important to realize that blood pressure is not a constant but a variable factor, depending on a number of conditions, especially nervous tension. As a matter of fact, sensitive people, without being aware of it, may be so tense about the results of the check-up that their pressure goes up. Others suffering some minor disorder may fear that they are seriously ill, and their pressure will go up. Still others have a family history of high blood pressure. All of them want to know whether reasons for fear exist, and therefore look at the checking of their pressure as a sort of oracle. In those cases the doctor is not surprised if the first reading is somewhat high. He knows that this "office visit hypertension" is bound to go down after the patient has calmed down and relaxed.

Office visit hypertension

The blood pressure of an otherwise healthy person can also go up in situations of more sustained tension and excitement, such as job or family problems, the death of someone close, before important school exams, etc. Once these conflicts have been resolved or adjusted to, the blood pressure returns to normal, as the following case demonstrates.

45

Repeated blood pressure readings of a middle-aged, seemingly depressed patient showed moderately elevated levels. Conversations with him revealed that he was married to a woman many years his junior. The couple had two children and now the once happy marriage was falling apart. The man was extremely upset over this. After his initial visit the doctor did not see the man for some time. A year later, after his divorce, the patient returned for a check-up. He said that he had gotten over the divorce and was able to visit his children regularly. His blood pressure was back to normal and has remained normal since.

Temporary elevations of blood pressure can also be brought on by some acute diseases, particularly of the kidneys, or by complications in pregnancy, and metabolic as well as nervous disorders.

Another important item, one of particular interest to

*Blood pres-
sure and the
Pill*

women, concerns drugs, among them oral contraceptives that can raise blood pressure to undesirably high levels. Anywhere from 15-20% of all women taking the Pill show a slight increase in pressure well within the normal range. But in some instances, although the exact percentage is not known, there is clear evidence of hypertension. As a rule, the pressure goes down again a few weeks after discontinuing the drug. Women who take contraceptive pills regularly should have their blood pressure checked frequently, particularly during the first few months. (For more detailed information on this see the section on high blood pressure, contraception, and pregnancy, p. 114.)

Among rarer drugs which, if taken in large quantities, may cause high blood pressure are licorice derivatives prescribed for some cases of peptic and duodenal ulcers. If you are taking such drugs don't be surprised if your doctor checks your blood pressure more frequently than usual.

To return to the initial question, what does high blood pressure mean? First, it can be a generally harmless symptom accompanying various psychological or physical disorders, harmless especially where the crucial factor responsible for cardiovascular complications—

permanence—is absent. But an elevated blood pressure level—as the subsequent chapters will make amply clear—can also be a serious symptom of an organic or nervous disease coupled with a permanent, and in the long run dangerous, disturbance of the pressure-regulator mechanism.

Blood Pressure and Old Age

ystolic pres-
ure increase
after 60

Many persons, in particular women, show a marked increase in their systolic pressure, frequently well above 160, after reaching the age of sixty, while their diastolic pressure remains normal. Their pressure range—between systolic and diastolic—is very wide. This age-related condition is not genuine hypertension but the by-product of arteriosclerotic deterioration of the major arteries, especially the aorta, and the resultant loss of elasticity. As these arteries harden and become more rigid they lose their adaptability. The walls, now inelastic, can no longer convert the blood output of the heart into a smoothly flowing stream. The result is an unbroken pulse wave with high (systolic) peaks and low (diastolic) valleys. Here, in contrast to genuine hypertensive disease, arteriosclerosis is the cause rather than the effect of elevated blood pressure. Persons suffering from this type of circulatory disorder frequently also have diabetes, abnormal fat metabolism, are heavy smokers, and show other risk factors related to arteriosclerosis.

Arterio-
sclerosis is
cause, not
effect

If their pressure does not exceed 170 mm Hg, and in the absence of other risk factors, the life expectancy of these persons is more or less normal. If, however, their readings are higher, the increased pressure may bring on congestive heart failure (see p. 53). In the case of advanced arteriosclerosis, just as in the case of chronic hypertension, there exists the danger of one or more typical complications. (See section on the consequences of hypertension, p. 53.)

47

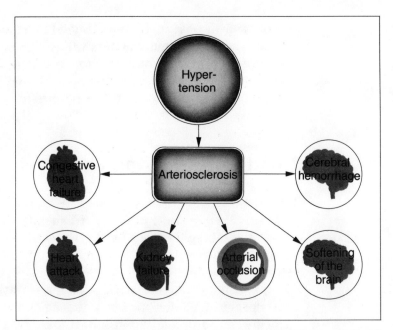

Injuries to the organ resulting from hypertension. The majority of these diseases are caused by an arteriosclerosis. Its development is strengthened and hastened by chronic high blood pressure.

Chronic High Blood Pressure (Hypertension)

Hypertension defined

Medical science defines hypertension as a chronic (i.e., slowly progressing, persistent) increase in the systolic and diastolic arterial blood pressure which can be caused by a variety of factors, but regardless of the cause follows a typical pattern. Two aspects of the disease represent potentially serious dangers: one, the tendency of the pressure to continue to rise and two, the resultant damage to the arteries, heart, brain, and kidneys. In this respect chronic hypertension differs from the less serious types of elevated pressure previously mentioned.

Chronic hypertension usually begins "silently," as a

48

rule after the age of thirty or forty. In certain exceptional cases it can begin quite early in life. In its initial stages, the pressure may go up only intermittently, as for example in situations of ordinary stress, such as long drives, and return to normal more slowly than usual. Or the pressure may go up only at work, not while resting or vacationing. In such cases we speak of a "labile hypertension," or if the readings lie in the upper normal range, of a "borderline hypertension." However, if the readings are consistently above normal, the disease has progressed to the "stable" stage.

Labile and stable hypertension

Chronic hypertension can take a variety of forms, examples of which abound. Every hospital knows of even young people with extremely high blood pressure, from 200/120 to 250/140. They are admitted with chief complaints of a feeling of general malaise, severe headaches, eye problems, and heart troubles. And their pressure does not go down significantly even after protracted bed rest. In cases like this we are probably dealing with a particularly aggressive type of hypertensive disease known as "malignant hypertension." It is called malignant because it progresses rapidly and dramatically and causes serious and early damage to the heart, brain, kidneys and eyes. Until fairly recently the prognosis for people with malignant hypertension was not very promising. Today their chances are considerably better. Because of early detection and treatment many cases of hypertension can be arrested before they become malignant. And even where the disease has progressed to that serious stage the pressure can often be reduced and brought down to less hazardous levels.

Malignant hypertension

In the majority of cases, chronic high blood pressure if treated can be brought down and its complications avoided. At least 95% of all hypertensives have a benign form of hypertension. That is to say, its progress is slower and its effects do not manifest themselves as early. Still, even the so-called "benign" type of hypertension is a danger to health and life.

Most cases are controllable

49

If your blood pressure is too high please keep in mind that no form of high blood pressure is really benign. Every sustained increase in your pressure, however slight, can mean the beginning of a disabling disease. You can prevent this from happening if your hypertension is detected in time and you follow your doctor's orders.

How High Blood Pressure Originates

The clinical picture of chronic hypertension—its symptoms, course, and complications—is quite clear but its causal factors and precipitating mechanisms cover a broad range. By causal factors we mean organic diseases; by precipitating mechanisms we mean personal habits and external influences that may foster the development of high blood pressure. It is essential that we distinguish between these two sets of circumstances. Whereas the causal agents are as a rule hereditary and appear spontaneously, the precipitating mechanisms can be controlled and eliminated.

Causal factors

Unfortunately we can identify only those causal factors with observable effects and which are linked to organic disease. The most common are inflammatory diseases of the kidneys, the various types of nephritis. But we know next to nothing about how and why they are linked to hypertension. We know a little more about the relationship between high blood pressure and various conditions that narrow the arteries of the kidneys (renal atrophy, hypoplasia, renal artery stenosis), thereby diminshing the blood supply to the kidneys and raising the blood pressure. It is possible that an increased production of a hormone-like substance, called renin by the defective

kidneys provokes the onset of hypertension. The type of
hypertension induced by kidney disease accounts for
about 15% of all cases of chronic high blood pressure.

Among the rare causal factors are tumors—generally
benign—of the adrenal glands, small organs about 2 inches
in length lying above the kidneys. They consist of two
layers that produce hormones essential to the circulatory
and metabolic functions of the body: the inner part
(medulla) produces noradrenaline and adrenaline, which
raise the blood pressure, and the outer part (cortex)
secretes hydrocortisone and aldosterone which—
indirectly—participate in the control of blood pressure.
Tumors can stimulate the adrenals to excessive hormonal
activity, which in turn can elevate the blood pressure to
abnormally high levels. The incidence of this type of
hypertension is low, about 1-2% of all cases. Another and
highly infrequent type of hypertension is caused by a
constriction of the aorta, the major artery leading from the
heart (aortic coarctation).

These organically caused types of high blood pressure
are referred to as "secondary hypertension," and they
account for only about 16-18% of all known cases of high
blood pressure. But in the overwhelming majority of all
known cases no such causal factors exist. We refer to
these as "primary" or "essential" hypertension.

Essential hypertension is a puzzling disease whose
causes and nature are still largely unexplored. Put in its
simplest form, it is a functional disorder of the nervous
circuit controlling blood pressure (see p. 39). But despite
intensive research we have not yet discovered the site of
the defect—whether the pressure-sensitive receptors send
out wrong information, whether the circulation center
itself is defective and overstimulates the sympathico-
adrenergic system, or whether the artery walls are unduly
sensitized and react abnormally. All these questions
remain unanswered.

A variety of factors, many unknown, apparently play a
part in this puzzling malfunction of blood pressure

Heredity plays an important role

regulation. We know that heredity plays an important role, as evidenced by the high incidence of essential hypertension running in families. Case histories show that the incidence of hypertension is greater among persons whose parents and grandparents suffered from high blood pressure or died of complications arising from it than among persons without a similar family history. Medical science knows next to nothing about the nature of this hereditary factor.

Precipitating mechanisms

We know a great deal more about the environmental influences that can set off and accelerate both primary and secondary hypertension. They are: obesity, a high-sodium diet, and, possibly, prolonged psychological stress.

Overweight

Excessive weight can enhance other risk factors and constitutes a serious health hazard. It is the crucial and at the same time most avoidable single known factor contributing to the development of high blood pressure. This was borne out emphatically by the Framingham study, which showed that persons whose weight was 20% above the norm run three times the risk of developing high blood pressure than those of normal weight. While the risk of hypertension increases with the amount of excess weight, weight loss can lower the pressure or even bring it down to normal.

Salt

Salt—the chemical sodium chloride—is an essential mineral required by the body. Whether salt is harmful to a person depends on his state of health and on how much salt he or she consumes. Ancient man, being a hunter and predator, lived on a low-salt diet, as do animals to this day. But as he learned to extract salt from the ocean and the earth he began to add it to his food. Salt became a seasoning in the preservation of meat and fish, and finally a major ingredient of our daily diet. The daily per capita salt consumption of Western man amounts to about ⅓-½ oz. (10-15g) whereas all we require is about ¹/₆ oz. (3-5g).

Animal experiments have shown that salt can in fact help raise our blood pressure. Among Eskimos, who eat very little salt, high blood pressure and stroke are very rare, while the Japanese, who are large salt consumers, have a high incidence of both. We also know that high salt intake can intensify an existing tendency toward hypertension while a low-salt diet can help keep it under control, as do certain drugs, the so-called diuretics, which stimulate the excretion of salt and are important in the treatment of the disease. The mechanism by which salt raises blood pressure is still unknown. All we know is that sodium plays the decisive role. Perhaps it is the content and distribution of sodium in the wall of the arteries that affects their sensitivity to sympathico-adrenergic stimulation.

Let us return briefly to the stress factor touched on earlier. According to a widely held belief tensions of all sorts can trigger high blood pressure. Job worries, social status, noise, aggression, agitation, anxiety, all these negative influences and emotions are thought to precipitate hypertension. But we have no definite proof that they do. What we do know is that they can raise the blood pressure temporarily and exacerbate existing hypertension. In some instances they can even turn "benign" hypertension into malignant hypertension. Even though conclusive evidence is still lacking we can safely assume that given a tendency toward hypertension—and only then—can frequent and prolonged stress facilitate and accelerate hypertension.

The Long-term Effects and Complications of Chronic Hypertension

The effects and complications of hypertension can be

divided into two categories: direct and indirect. In the vast majority of cases the direct consequences—congestive heart failure and cerebral hemorrhage (stroke)—can be prevented if the pressure is brought down to and maintained at normal levels.

The left heart ventricle of an untreated hypertensive patient must labor against increased arterial resistance. For a while the heart muscle can adjust to this increased

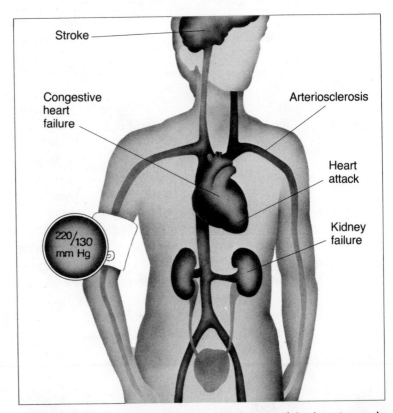

Damage caused by hypertension. Weakness of the heart muscle, calcification of the arteries (arteriosclerosis), stroke (cerebral), cardiac infarction, kidney failure. To a large extent, these dangerous complications caused by hypertension can be avoided if the disease is recognized early and properly treated.

burden by becoming bigger (left ventricular hypertrophy), similar to the muscles of an athlete in training. But if the high pressure persists the demands on the heart will exceed its capacity to adapt and work efficiently. The muscle fibers will slacken, and the end result is the dilation and ultimate collapse of the left ventricle (left ventricular insufficiency). When the disabled left heart can no longer accomodate the flow of pulmonary blood, the blood is backed up into the lungs. If left untreated this pulmonary congestion can overburden and ultimately paralyze the right ventricle as well (right ventricular insufficiency). When that happens, the uptake of venous blood by the heart is diminished and the legs retain fluid, a condition *Edema* known as edema.

The cerebral arteries (of the brain) are particularly subject to the burden of elevated pressure. Under the prolonged mechanical overload tiny blisters, so-called aneurysms, can form along the walls of the arteries. With a sudden increase in blood pressure, as for example under conditions of emotional or physical strain, these blisters can burst, and the blood gushing out can destroy or paralyze adjacent brain tissue (stroke).

All other complications are of an indirect nature, i.e., *Indirect con-* they are not the immediate result of the increased pressure *sequences* but of premature and severe arteriosclerosis evoked by chronic hypertension. The areas most likely to suffer long-term ill effects are the coronary and brain arteries.

The coronary arteries, the "lifeline" supplying the vital oxygen, are the vessels threatened the most. Because they are comparatively narrow, arteriosclerotic obstruction, popularly referred to as hardening of the coronary arteries, can seriously interfere with the blood flow to the heart muscle. This insufficient coronary perfusion will manifest itself whenever the heart's demand for oxygen and energy exceeds the limited supply the constricted vessels allow to pass through. This may happen under the most ordinary circumstances—while climbing stairs, during bowel movement, while excited. The heart muscle responds to

55

the curtailed blood supply with typical symptoms as oppression or pain in the left chest which can radiate to

the left shoulder and arm. The medical name for these complaints is angina pectoris (Latin for chest constriction). Chronic blood and oxygen deficiency of the heart muscle can gradually destroy the myocardial muscle fibers (muscle degeneration). Eventually this will result in congestive heart failure, often preceded by arrhythmia—irregular heart beat.

Angina pectoris frequently is the forerunner of the total occlusion of the coronary artery. When that happens the muscle tissue previously supplied by the blocked artery dies. The result is a myocardial infarct—a heart attack—the most serious and dangerous catastrophe that can happen in the heart. Even now almost 40% of all persons

who have a heart attack die within the first few days, many of them before they can even be rushed to the hospital.

And like the heart, the brain too may suffer serious damage if arteriosclerosis obstructs its blood supply. The result is the slow degeneration of brain tissue popularly known as "softening of the brain." Cerebral infarction (the sudden occlusion of a brain artery) as a rule is less severe than a cerebral hemorrhage and its symptoms (paralysis, aphasia) respond more readily to treatment.

Arteriosclerotic obstructions are not confined to the coronary and brain vessels. They can occur in other blood vessels of the body as well. Hypertensives who smoke heavily can develop severe obstructions of the pelvic and leg arteries which make walking difficult and cause

intermittent limping. Cigarette smoking in particular seems to affect the circulation in the legs.

Hypertension is particularly damaging to the sensitive arteries and arterioles (the smallest muscle arteries) of the kidneys. One might even say that every chronic case of hypertension, regardless of its origin, sooner or later will result in sclerosis and obstruction of the kidney arteries and arterioles. In its most severe form this can result in kidney failure and in the poisoning of the body by

Uremia　metabolic wastes which the kidneys are unable to eliminate, a condition known as uremia. A once invariable fatal condition, uremia today has lost much of its terror. Artificial kidney machines and other advances in the treatment of kidney disease have given the victims of this once dreaded disease a new lease on life.

4. How to Recognize High Blood Pressure

When we become ill our body usually sends out signals. We refer to them as symptoms. For example, when our respiratory tract becomes infected we respond by coughing and perhaps run a temperature. A duodenal ulcer announces itself by pain and heartburn. Medical literature lists thousands of such warning signals by which the body notifies us that something has gone wrong. Unfortunately, high blood pressure sends us no such warnings. It can frequently persist for many years undetected and un-treated. That is why it is often referred to as the silent disease or "silent killer." There are no typical symptoms or signs. By looking at a person it is impossible to say whether he does or does not suffer from high blood pressure. In the early stages of the disease the patient usually feels quite healthy and happy. If there are any complaints they are not necessarily those one might associate with hypertension.

The silent killer

We can differentiate between two categories of com-plaints and symptoms, and they are related to the length and severity of the disease.

Complaints and Symptoms

1. Non-specific symptoms before any complications of hypertension have set in.

• The following list of complaints are those most frequently mentioned by persons suffering from *prolonged cases of hypertension*. But since they appear just as frequently in persons of the same age group who do not have high blood pressure, they can also be symptomatic of other disorders.

Non-specific complaints in hypertension

Complaint	Frequency (approx.)
Nervousness	35%
Palpitation	32%
Dizziness	30%
Chest pain	26%
Headaches	23%
Depression, lack of drive	7%

Nervous im-balance

• *The patient with "nervous instability."* By this we mean an imbalance of the autonomic nervous system (p. 39), which reacts more labile and more strongly than either required or useful. Younger people with "labile hypertension" often have one or more symptom of nervous instability varying in degree and frequency. They include excessive perspiration, digestive and sleeping problems, fatigue, and excitability. Yet they are not necessarily typical of high blood pressure. Many persons with normal blood pressure have exactly the same symptoms. In some instances the sympathetic nervous system (see p. 39) can go into such high gear that cardiovascular complaints will completely dominate the clinical picture.

The older person with "functional deficiency." **Men** above
the age of forty-five years suffering from hypertension
often complain of not functioning at their best. They do

*Poor job
performance*

not perform as well on their jobs, they cannot handle
stresses and strains as well as before, they tire more
easily, their memory and concentration declines, their
sexual drive diminishes. Women in this age group have the
additional factor of menopause to cope with.

*2. Warning signals of high blood pressure where compli-
cations have already set in.* Many people with hypertension do not seek medical help until some of the
complications have set in. Only then do they find out that
they have high blood pressure.
Here are some of the typical complaints:

• *Incipient cardiac failure.* The first indications are short-
ness of breath after minimal exertion, often also a
persistent cough (pulmonary congestion) as well as
urination at night (which may also have other causes.) A
more specific symptom of congestive heart failure is
swelling of the ankles (so-called edema) at first only during
the day, not at night (which explains the urge to urinate)
but later turns into a permanent condition involving both
lower and upper legs.
• *Insufficient blood flow through the coronary vessels.*
Angina pectoris-like pains induced by excitement or stress
(see p. 56): tightness in the chest, pressure and pain
possibly radiating to the neck, the left shoulder, left arm
and left hand.
• *Insufficient blood flow to the cerebral arteries.* Non-
specific early symptoms such as dizziness, memory lapses,
inability to concentrate are followed by typical symptoms
of intermittent blood shortage in various sections of the
brain: fainting, temporary speech problems, difficulties
with walking, intermittent weakness of arms and/or legs.

• *Partial obstruction of the pelvic and leg arteries.*
Symptoms are leg cramps while walking (intermittent),
usually in one leg, rarely in both. As time goes on, the
distance a person is able to walk without frequent rest
stops becomes progressively shorter. In Europe this is
called the "window-shopper's" disease, because the
patient needs to stand still before the cramp disappears
and he can resume walking.

Rare signs Occasionally a patient may experience atypical though
very disturbing "circulatory attacks," accompanied by
palpitation, excessive perspiration, pallor, anxiety, weakness, and vague feelings of discomfort in the region of the
heart, all of this triggered by a sudden surge of extremely
high pressure. Such sudden attacks may signify a
condition known as pheochromocytoma (see p. 51), which
stimulates the release of vast quantities of adrenal
hormones into the blood stream. Attacks of this type are
warning signals of a rare and dangerous but operable type
of hypertension.

Some Important Indicators

Even though hypertension does not manifest itself through
typical symptoms, important indications of its possible
presence nonetheless do exist.

• The family history
• The personal history

Heredity Try to find out whether any members of your immediate
family have had hypertension, since heredity is a major
factor in essential hypertension, the most common type of
high blood pressure (see p. 52). It may not always be easy
to find out whether your parents' or grandparents'
immediate families have a history of high blood pressure.

62

If you cannot get this information try to learn whether anyone in their families had strokes, congestive heart failure or died of heart attacks—the most common complications of hypertension. These can be important clues to the existence of a hereditary disposition. It would also be important to know whether your family has a history of such crucial risk factors as diabetes, hyper-cholesterolemia, or gout.

One important warning sign of your personal history is long-standing overweight, especially if you were thin when young and put on anywhere from 30 to 40 pounds or more since then. If that is the case you are a high hypertension risk. Other warning signals are not quite so obvious. As mentioned earlier, kidney disease and hypertension often go hand in hand. Sometimes the patient doesn't even know that his kidneys are affected. Chronic tonsillitis in childhood can be a forerunner of kidney disease. Long-forgotten kidney infections, so-called "harmless" bladder irritations or kidney stones may indicate kidney disease that could lead to high blood pressure.

Long-standing overweight

A checklist of complaints, symptoms and indicators

1. Do you know whether members of your immediate family (parents, grandparents, brothers, sisters) have or have had high blood pressure?
   a. One member?
   b. More than one?

2. Did any member of your immediate family have or die of:
   a. Stroke
   b. Heart attack
   c. Congestive heart failure
   d. Kidney failure

3. Do or did you have a kidney disease?
   a. Did you often have tonsillitis?
   b. Were albumin (protein) and/or red blood cells ever found in your urine?
   c. Have you ever had a kidney infection or frequent "bladder irritations"?

4. Do you suffer from
   a. Nervousness
   b. Palpitations, chest pain
   c. Frequent headaches
   d. Dizziness
   e. Shortage of breath after physical exertion

5. Are you overweight?
   a. What is your normal weight?
   b. Does your weight exceed your normal weight by 10% or perhaps even 20%?

6. Do you believe that you are subjected to severe psychological stress?

Your answers to this check list give valuable information about your family and personal health profile. Discuss it with your doctor.

5. The Diagnostic Program

If you are found to have high blood pressure your doctor
will schedule a series of additional examinations. You may
question his advice but after you read the section on the
possible complications of hypertension (see p. 53) you will
understand his reasons. These tests and examinations
serve several purposes:
1. to determine the extent of the hypertensive disease,
2. to find its cause,

Purpose of
tests
3. to search for additional risk factors.

Determining the Extent of the Disease

he first step

The first objective of the diagnostic program is to deter-
mine exactly how far the disease has progressed, whether
the hypertension is malignant or not (see p. 49), whether
the arteries and internal organs have been affected, etc.
Your doctor has to know all this before he can draw up
your treatment program. The section on the general
check-up (see p. 69) tells you how your doctor proceeds.

67

Isolating the Cause

The second objective of the diagnostic program is to isolate the specific cause. We already know that high blood pressure can be caused by a variety of factors (see p. 50). Its diagnosis is a matter of elimination. That is to say, your doctor, before making a diagnosis of essential or primary hypertension, will dismiss the possibility of secondary hypertension only after checking you for all the organic diseases known to cause high blood pressure. Some of these hypertensive conditions such as unilateral atrophic kidney disease, renal artery stenosis, coarctation of the aorta, adrenal tumors, etc., can be cured by surgery. They are very rare, accounting for no more than about 4-5% of the total known cases of hypertension, but their early detection can make the difference between a normal life and premature death.

Kidney infection

A somewhat larger number, about 10%, is caused by kidney infections that respond to antibacterial or other drug therapy. An elevated blood pressure level frequently is the only indication of a kidney disease which, if left untreated, could result in kidney failure and death. Its detection is of immense importance not only for the treatment of hypertension but for the treatment of a potentially fatal kidney disease.

A process of elimination

The Search for Additional Risk Factors

Another vitally important aspect of the examination, the search for additional risk factors, should not be neglected, unless you have recently had a complete physical check-up.

68

The Basic Examination

Once the physician has diagnosed high blood pressure he
will suggest a series of tests to guide him in setting up your
treatment plan. General practitioners, cardiologists,
radiologists, and researchers have been debating the best
and most promising approach to such a broad-spectrum
examination, one that will isolate all possible causes of
secondary hypertension and check all possible organ
damage. Still, the scope of this examination should not
exceed the capability of your local doctor nor should it be
too costly.

Thorough
checkup

What do you expect your doctor to do in a complete
physical examination? The doctor will inquire into the
incidence of high blood pressure, heart attacks, stroke,
diabetes, obesity, gout, kidney disease in your family, ask
you about diseases you have had, about medication you
are taking, about stress in your work and life situation.
Your answers can furnish important diagnostic clues. If
you have specific complaints and pains try to describe
them as precisely as you can: the type and site of the pain,
its frequency, what foods or weather conditions seem to
trigger it, etc. All such information may prove to be
important. Tell your doctor about your general physical
and mental state, your diminished capabilities, if any, your
difficulties in concentration, and memory lapses, if any. To
evaluate your past history your doctor must know
something about your personal life. That is why he will ask
questions about your eating, smoking and drinking habits,
your work situation, your marriage and family life, the
physical activity you engage in, and how you spend your
leisure.

The physical examination begins with a thorough check
of your cardiovascular system. He listens for the
frequency and regularity of the heart beat (60-80 beats per
minutes are the norm) and for cardiac murmurs that might
indicate defects of the heart valves and he looks for
arrhythmias and premature beats symptomatic of·a

Check of the
cardio-
vascular
system

69

damaged heart muscle. He auscultates the lungs for signs of congestion related to the heart (p. 32). In checking this he may of course discover other pulmonary or bronchial disorders like a chronic smoker's bronchitis or emphysema which put an extra burden on the heart. Finally he palpates the big arteries at the neck, wrist, groin, and feet to test whether a pulse can be felt and whether it is strong or weak. A faint or nonexistent pulse at any of these sites is a warning sign of a developing arteriosclerotic obstruction (p. 56). Pain in the kidney region may point to a kidney disease which in the absence of any other symptoms might have gone undetected.

Laboratory tests The laboratory tests are designed to help detect the cause of hypertension. A high albumin (protein) and/or red blood cell content in the urine point to kidney infection. A high creatinine blood level (creatinine is a metabolic waste excreted in the urine) points to impaired kidney function. A low potassium level may be due to medication, but it may also point to adrenal-caused hypertension.

If your blood pressure remains high, particularly if you are no longer young, and the diastolic level stays above 100, your doctor is certain to order further tests.

EKG Few people really know how the electrocardiogram (EKG) works. To put it simply, the EKG is a continuous recording of the bioelectrical impulses (see p. 34) that stimulate and regulate heart activity. Deviations from the curve plotted by the highly sensitive apparatus can indicate either arrhythmias, changes in the heart muscle due to high pressure, impaired blood flow through the coronary vessels, or other irregularities and defects.

The chest X-ray (the amount of radiation involved is minimal and hence, harmless) yields additional information about the heart and lungs; whether the heart is enlarged or the lungs congested or whether the aorta shows signs of arteriosclerotic deterioration.

The kidney X-ray (pyelogram), which also takes in the renal pelvis and ureter, can detect chronic infections,

70

kidney stones, atrophied kidneys, or other defects which even though asymptomatic may still be the cause of hypertension.

The eyes   Don't be surprised if your doctor examines your eyes or refers you to an opthalmologist, for the condition of the retina (eyeground) and its small arteries are important diagnostic indicators. The eye more than any other single organ can show whether hypertension is becoming malignant (see p. 49). If so he may recommend hospitalization, additional diagnostic tests and initiate prompt treatment.

Special Tests

If secondary hypertension is suspected, all the possible causes must be checked out. For example, a sudden rise in blood pressure may be a sign of pheochromocytoma (see p. 62), or an abnormally low potassium level may point to a tumor of the adrenal cortex. Further tests are needed to find out whether excessive amounts of their specific hormones are being excreted in the urine or have been accumulated in the blood. Once this has been established the site of the tumor can be explored. A special X-ray technique (angiography) involving the injection of a dye is used to visualize the network of the aorta, the renal and adrenal arteries. Angiography may also be used where renal artery stenosis, an atrophied kidney or some other operable cause of hypertension is suspected.

Additional   Additional examinations may be needed to evaluate the
aminations   extent of the hypertensive damage discovered in the course of the general check-up. Angiography can show dangerous arteriosclerotic obstructions of the carotid, coronary, pelvic and leg arteries and indicate the advisability of surgery. Or neurological examinations may be needed to determine the extent of arterial brain damage. Testing the sensory and peripheral nerves (see p.

28) with an electroencephalography (EEG)—something like the EKG—as well as ultrasonic examinations and similar sophisticated techniques give surprisingly accurate pictures of the condition of various parts of the brain.

These secondary forms of hypertension are very rare, so the chances that one of them is the cause of your high blood pressure are minimal. Yet, if it were so, you could consider yourself quite lucky because they are operable. Likewise, if the examination reveals that you have an unsuspected kidney disease this can be successfully treated. In all these cases early detection and correct diagnosis are prerequisites for successful treatment and cure.

In case you are concerned about the safety of diagnostic techniques like X-ray or kidney tests involving radioactive substances, let me point out: all of them are tested, safe, routine procedures, and most of them need be done only once. The minor pain or discomfort caused by the insertion of the angiogram needle can be avoided with a local anesthetic.

The Doctor-Patient Talk

What are the expectations of the doctor and of the patient?
• *The patient* wants to learn the results, to understand them, and to be told clearly what the treatment involves.
• *The doctor* wants the patient to be interested and cooperative.

What each expects

Whether their expectations are fulfilled depends largely on their talk following the test results. Doctors attach great importance to this conference.

You must learn to overcome your reluctance to ask questions, and you must keep on asking until you understand the findings and their consequences. That may not be as easy as it sounds. Don't be afraid of wasting your doctor's valuable time or that he may think you are slow if you don't understand a complicated medical problem right away. That would be wrong. Doctors know how difficult it is for laymen to understand medical terms or problems and they want to help.

6. How to Succeed in the Treatment of High Blood Pressure

Enormous advances

In recent years medicine has made enormous strides in the treatment of high blood pressure. Attitudes and approaches have changed. In the past doctors tended to play down the potential dangers. Because there were no overt symptoms in the earlier stages, fatal strokes or heart attacks were considered accidents of fate rather than the consequences of persistent hypertension. At the same time they were fatalistic because there was no effective treatment for the disease and its attendant problems until the early '60s.

Drug treatment

Today we know that in untreated hypertension life expectancy is inversely proportional to the level of blood pressure. But we also have drugs that will control almost every type of hypertension and bring the pressure down to safe levels. This in most cases means a substantial increase in life expectancy and an improvement in the quality of life.

Figures that speak for themselves

Having read the foregoing chapters you know that treatment is of vital importance. But perhaps you are one

75

of those skeptics who need proof, who want the hard facts on which we base our optimistic prognosis.

Optimistic statistics

• **Stroke.** In the past at least 20%, and according to some statistics, as many as 30-35% of all hypertensives had fatal strokes. Today the incidence is no higher than among persons with normal blood pressure.

• **Congestive heart failure.** Before the discovery of effective treatment almost 75% of all persons who died of congestive heart failure (CHF) had high blood pressure. The average life expectancy after the onset of CHF was 2 to 5 years. Today death from CHF is rare in treated cases of hypertension.

• **Heart attack.** At first glance the statistics here do not look quite so good. The incidence of heart attacks apparently has remained the same. Why has treatment not been effective? Or is it possible that hypertension is not a risk factor in heart attacks?

Statistics may be confusing

The answer is not all that simple and the total picture is somewhat more favorable than would seem at first glance. What the statistics fail to show is that persons who are treated for hypertension live longer then they did when fatal complications were more common; without treatment they might well have died of a heart attack at the age of 49 instead of at age 69. In other words the statistics do not take the greater life expectancy into account. Moreover, people with high blood pressure are likely to have other coronary risk factors (see p. 16). So if they have a heart attack even though their pressure has been normalized one will have to ask whether they perhaps suffer from hypercholesterolemia, smoke cigarettes, are diabetic—any one or a combination of all of these may be responsible. It is the conviction of all epidemiologists and clinicians that the heart attack incidence among hypertensives will decrease substantially with the early detection and treatment of any and all risk factors.

Individual Treatment Plans and Methods

Various approaches

The decision when to begin treatment and what kind of drugs to use depends on many individual factors—the patient's age, whether his hypertension is labile or stable, benign or malignant, etc. Different conditions call for different approaches. Some patients need immediate medication, others don't. The fact that different patients receive different treatment can cause misunderstandings which should be cleared up. It is not unusual to hear a patient complain that his doctor didn't start him on the right medication or that he overmedicated him. Isn't it odd that people who would never question the expertise of the auto mechanic who repairs their car, will not hestitate to second-guess their doctor.

One of the reasons this book was written was to clear up misconceptions and misunderstandings. Let us look at some hypothetical cases to show why doctors prescribe different treatments for different people.

Three examples

The first example concerns a young man with signs of nervous lability (see p. 49) with intermittent elevation of his blood pressure and a non-contributing personal and family history. Experience has shown that this "borderline hypertension" can disappear in the course of time, yet it can also develop into chronic hypertension. Therefore the doctor will not upset the patient by putting him on a permanent regime of medication—with its possible side effects—before monitoring his blood pressure over a longer period of time.

The second example is that of a young man with a slight but constant increase in blood pressure. On his father's side there is a family history of hypertension, heart attack, and stroke. In this case the insignificant elevation of the blood pressure may well herald chronic hypertension. Therefore the doctor decides on a different course of treatment. He will try to normalize the pressure with

77

medication to prevent possible damage to the heart and
circulation and he will try to eliminate other risk factors.

The third example involves a patient in his sixties
suffering from adult-onset diabetes, high blood fat level,
and a moderately high systolic pressure, in the 170-180
range. The diastolic pressure was and has remained
normal. This type of systolic pressure increase (see p. 47)
is the result of arteriosclerosis, which in turn is the result
of this patient's risk factors. In this case antihypertensive
drugs are not indicated as long as the systolic pressure
does not go up any further, for they can neither cure his
arteriosclerosis nor increase his life expectancy.

Doctor-Patient Cooperation

Professor G. von Bergmann, a philosopher among
clinicians, has stated that the successful treatment of
chronic diseases requires two strong personalities: the

Two strong
personalities
needed

doctor and the patient. What he obviously meant by this is
that chronic diseases demand "chronic" treatment, and
that the success of long-range therapy depends not only on
medication but also on personality factors. The doctor's
efforts on behalf of a patient can be successful only if they
meet with understanding, cooperation, and disciplined
adherence to his orders.

7. The Doctor's Role

Long-range Drug Therapy

A patient with high blood pressure is likely to ask the doctor how much his pressure has to go down before he can stop worrying, whether he can discontinue the medication once the pressure has been normalized, and whether he must take all the pills his doctor has prescribed.

The objective in the treatment of hypertension is to bring down the pressure—particularly the diastolic reading—to a level appropriate to the patient's age (see p. 26). Those patients who present problems usually show arteriosclerotic damage in one or more of the arteries leading to the vital organs. Bringing down the pressure too abruptly can interfere with the flow of blood to the brain, resulting in vertigo and dizziness, or interfere with the flow of blood to the kidneys. But most patients respond well to

Gradual lowering of pressure

the lowering of the pressure if it is done gradually and carefully over a period of weeks rather than days. In serious cases with major arteriosclerotic complications—where the blood pressure cannot be brought down to the level appropriate to the patient's age it can usually be brought to somewhat less dangerous ranges. Hypertension that does not respond to treatment at all is extremely rare, a fact all those who suffer from the disease should find very reassuring.

79

Concerning the question of how long treatment must continue, the answer is: forever. Secondary hypertension

which can be cured through surgery is rare. *In all other types of hypertension medication can only eliminate the symptoms; it cannot cure its underlying cause.* The body apparently is not able to learn how to correct the chronic disturbance of the regulatory mechanism. The blood pressure cannot return to normal levels without outside help. Every interruption of the treatment therefore means an almost immediate rise in blood pressure. Medication becomes a lifelong companion in the maintenance of normal or tolerable pressure levels, like insulin in the case of diabetes or eyeglasses for people with poor vision. After all, taking pills regularly does not seem too high a price for the chance to lead an almost normal life.

The type and quantity of drugs prescribed in the treatment of hypertension vary from patient to patient. If the blood pressure is only moderately high the doctor may prescribe only a single drug, while in cases of serious hypertension he may prescribe a combination of drugs. These patients usually question both the number of pills they are told to take and the possible harmful side effects. The answer is that the prescription of two or more drugs serves a useful purpose. The drugs used in hypertension have to be "strong" to be effective, and in the long run such strong drugs may have undersirable side effects. If one would treat a severe case of hypertension with one single drug, one would by necessity have to increase its dosage. This could conceivably lead to a higher risk of side effects. However this can be avoided by utilizing a

combination therapy regime. Several antihypertensive drugs may be used simultaneously, all with different modes of action and, therefore, with different side effects.

Antihypertensive Drugs

Before discussing specific drugs I would like to cite some

very depressing figures: according to world-wide statistics only about 20% of all diagnosed hypertensives take the drugs prescribed for them. In other words, 80% of all people with high blood pressure fail to take advantage of the opportunity to stay healthier longer. This pattern is wasteful both in terms of money and health, and it will take a concerted educational campaign to overcome the resistance of patients to drugs.

Perhaps you are among the many who distrust and reject drugs. Perhaps you are afraid that they will do more harm than good. After all, we hear and read a lot about approved drugs which are later banned because prolonged use has produced unsuspected harmful effects. And the labels of all drugs contain long warnings about the possible adverse effects. However, the layman tends to overestimate both the frequency and seriousness of such adverse reactions. Still, many patients, unable to weigh the risk of side effects objectively, tend to overreact to these warnings.

One of the most important things I have learned in the course of my practice is that patients will adhere to a prescribed course of treatment more rigidly if they know what it is they are taking and why they are asked to take that specific drug. That holds true particularly for patients on long-term or permanent drug therapy. Once the reason for and the effects of the medication have been explained to them they turn from passive objects of treatment into interested allies in the fight against their disease.

That is why, despite all justified medical misgivings about "overinformation" and "medical half-knowledge," I have included a brief listing of drugs used to combat hypertension. The list is limited to drugs used in long-range treatment; it tells you how they work and their possible side effects. If and when these drugs should be taken by you and in what amounts, only your doctor can tell you.

Drugs that lower blood pressure by excretion of salt

Diuretics   Diuretics are drugs that excrete sodium through the
kidneys. That explains the great urge to urinate in the
initial phase of treatment. By decreasing the sodium
content of the body diuretics (indirectly) lower the blood
pressure. As you will recall sodium increases the blood
pressure of people with hypertension (see p. 52). By taking
diuretics regularly they can avoid going on a completely
salt-free diet. All they have to do is reduce their salt intake
$^1/_{10}$-$^1/_5$ oz. (3-5 g) daily. Diuretics not only get rid of excess
salt, they also have two additional important advantages:
• They enhance the effectiveness of other antihypertensive
medications, which means reduced dosages and therefore
fewer undesirable side effects.
• Because they stimulate salt and water excretion, they
help hypertensives with congestive heart failure to
eliminate their edema.

That is why diurectics are among the most frequently
used antihypertensive drugs. Doctors prefer diuretics with
long-lasting effects (8-18 hours or even 24-36 hours)
because they don't have to be taken more than once a day
or even only every 2 to 3 days.

Because the side effects of diurectics are unlike those of
any of the other antihypertensive drugs they will be
discussed here rather than together with those of the other
drugs (see p. 85). Considering their wide use the side
effects are comparatively rare, preventable on the whole,
and almost always of short duration. The most common
Drop in   one is a drop in the potassium level because they stimulate
potassium   the excretion of potassium along with sodium. The
level   consequences are generally minor and detectable only by
measuring the serum potassium level. A serious low
potassium level can cause arrhythmia, loss of appetite,
constipation, fatigue and muscle weakness, for the muscle
cells require large quantities of potassium. Severe drops in
the potassium level can turn a simple physical effort like

82

climbing stairs, getting up from a chair, or carrying a light package into a major task. So when your doctor asks you to have your potassium level checked you should listen to him. Foods rich in potassium and special potassium preparations can prevent or compensate for a lack of potassium. There is a growing tendency on the part of doctors to prescribe drugs that combine the properties of the diuretics with the capacity to inhibit potassium excretion.

Blood sugar and uric acid levels

In the course of your treatment it is likely that from time to time your doctor will check your blood sugar and uric acid levels. He does this for two reasons: in diabetics or persons with a tendency toward diabetes diuretics can affect the sugar metabolism and possibly raise the blood sugar level. And where there is a hereditary predisposition to gout the elevated uric acid level may go up, together with deposits or urate crystals in the joints, particularly the big toe. Those readers who have suffered attacks of gout know how painful that can be. Medications that depress the blood uric acid level can prevent this.

None of these conditions should cause serious concern. As soon as the patient is taken off diuretics the sugar and uric acid metabolism almost invariably returns to baseline levels.

Drugs that lower blood pressure levels directly

Rauwolfia derivatives

Certain drugs lower the blood pressure by directly acting on the regulatory mechanism that controls blood pressure (see p. 40). For a long time the rauwolfia derivatives, especially reserpine, were the most widely used drugs in hypertension therapy. They inhibit the activity of the sympathico-adrenergic system by eliminating part of the noradrenaline stored in the arterial walls (see p. 39). Rauwolfia derivatives work safely, slowly, and gently. They have a tranquilizing, pleasant effect. But if taken in large doses they can cause depressions; therefore some doctors are reluctant to prescribe them.

Recently a new group of drugs, the beta receptor
blockers, have come into increasing use. They act gently
and are effective, particularly in mild or moderate cases of
hypertension, particularly for patients with a hyperactive
sympathetic nervous system who have an increased pulse
rate and palpitations (see p. 60). Beta blockers are well
tolerated. Having said all this it is paradoxical to have to
tell you that they are counterindicated for a comparatively
large number of patients: those with congestive heart
failure, slow pulse, asthma, impaired peripheral arterial
circulation, and instable diabetes.

Beta
blockers

Hydralazine

Hydralazine, a well known antihypertensive drug, is
being used with increasing frequency since the introduc-
tion of the beta blockers. It has proved particularly
effective when used in combination with them, since the
antihypertensive properties of the two act jointly while
their undesirable side effects (acceleration of pulse rate
with hydralazine, slowing of pulse rate with beta blockers)
cancel each other. Hydralazine relaxes the musculature of
the arterial wall and thereby lowers flow resistance and
blood pressure. It should not be used alone where the
blood flow to the coronary arteries is impaired.

Methyldopa

The effectiveness of methyldopa rests on an ingenious
arrangement. Methyldopa is closely related to dopamine,
the basic component in the production of noradrenaline.
Methyldopa, when taken in large quantities, induces the
body's biochemical laboratories to produce methyl-
noradrenaline, its harmless derivative, instead of the
tension-inducing noradrenaline. Methyldopa is a moderately strong, slow-working drug that must be taken 2-4
times daily. It has few effects, but should not be
prescribed for persons with liver disease.

Clonidine

Clonidine is among the heavy artillery. It inhibits the
parts of sympathico-adrenergic system located in the
brain, which serves to lower arterial resistance and pulse
rate—and the blood pressure goes down. Its effects wear
off quickly and therefore it must be taken a few times

84

daily. Particular attention has to be paid to its side effects (see p. 87). *The sudden discontinuation of clonidine can cause serious problems.* For this reason one should never cut down on the dosage or discontinue taking it without first checking with your doctor.

uanethidine Guanethidine is one of the most powerful antihypertensive drugs. It works by blocking the transmission of impulses from the brain to the blood vessels. It is slow-acting and long-lasting. That is why doctors increase the dosage cautiously until the daily requirement is reached. As is to be expected in so powerful a drug undesirable and serious side effects are also more common, though not necessarily inevitable.

Side Effects.

If you are being treated with antihypertensive drugs don't miss this section.

Antihypertensive drugs produce two basically different groups of side effects which everyone on this type of medication should know about. On the one hand, comparatively minor discomfort which should not cause undue alarm, but on the other hand, warning signals of typical side effects that should be recognized and immediately brought to the attention of the doctor.

Initial discomfort

ypotensive symptoms In the early days or weeks of drug therapy some patients experience symptoms of low blood pressure (hypotension), the reason being that the brain, long accustomed to a pressure of let us say 200/120 mm Hg initially reacts to lowered levels of say 140/90 as though they were suffering from hypotension. This sensation persists until the brain has adjusted to the lower pressure.

85

If you are being treated with antihypertensive drugs you should know that such harmless reactions generally don't last more than a few weeks. During this transitional period patients frequently complain that everything seems slowed down: their thinking, their reactions, even their speech. Their concentration and memory are affected, work seems more difficult, they need more sleep.

Everything slows down

The patient may think that since the pills make him feel worse instead of better something must be wrong with the treatment. He may decide to cut down on the dosage or stop taking the drugs altogether without consulting his doctor. That would be a bad mistake and, beyond that, a dangerous and shortsighted course. These symptoms can be avoided or at least kept to a minimum by bringing down the pressure gradually over a period of two to three weeks.

There are, of course, exceptions. While some people have practically no problems, others respond with serious complaints for a long time. If the discomfort persists or if the reactions are very severe (drowsiness, nausea, vertigo) the doctor must be informed promptly. He can check to see whether the decrease in blood pressure has exceeded the tolerance of the brain or kidneys, i.e., whether these reactions are the results of "relative hypotension" or of an inability to tolerate the medication.

Specific side effects and their warning signals

This section does not deal with the minor, temporary reactions to the lowering of the blood pressure but with the typical side effects of specific drugs.

Practically all drugs have undesirable side effects. One might even say that there can be no effective drug against high blood pressure without some side effects. However, the extent and degree of the individual response to a given drug cannot be predicted. It is therefore essential that everyone taking any of these drugs learn about the possible side effects and their warning signals.

86

Excessive fatigue, dullness, weakness, and loss of energy can be caused by clonidine, reserpin, and to a lesser extent methyldopa as well. Patients on these medications must be prepared for these symptoms for they can become work and driving hazards. That is one of the reasons that I have devoted a section especially to the realtionship between hypertension and driving (see p. 113). Undesirable side effects can often be eliminated by reducing dosages; if that does not work other drugs may have to be substituted.

Work and driving hazards

Vertigo, dizziness, and a tendency to fall can be brought on by guanethidine and sometimes by other powerful antihypertensive drugs as well. Because these medications affect the sympathico-adrenergic system (p. 41) they can block the adaptive mechanisms of the circulation which prevent a sudden drop in blood pressure when getting up from a sitting position or when standing. To put it differently: guanethidine and occasionally methyldopa and clonidine will lower the blood pressure more in an upright position than when lying down. If the dosage taken is too large the pressure can go down so much as to cause fainting spells. A person treated with these drugs or someone who for any other reason reacts similarly should avoid excessive exposure to the sun, alcohol, rich foods, and strenuous physical activity. A patient experiencing any of these sensations should immediately inform his doctor.

Heart Drugs

Digitalis

A hypertensive patient with congestive heart failure usually takes digitalis. Digitalis eases the work of the heart muscle by increasing its ability to contract with less oxygen. The heart begins to beat more powerfully and more economically. Frequently digitalis alone will "regulate" the rapid, irregular heart beat, the arrhythmia (see p. 69) of some hypertensives. Digitalis is not habit-forming and never loses its effectiveness. In congestive heart failure it is quite literally a lifesaver which can safely be taken over a long period of time. In some cases hypertensives whose arrhythmias are the result of congestive heart failure (see p. 54) must also take

Arrhythmias   additional drugs. Arrhythmias must be treated if they constitute a hazard (for example, multiple extra beats), if they substantially impair the performance of the heart (too rapid or too slow pulse rate). Patients who suffer from frequent or constant arrhythmias should call this to their doctor's attention. He will decide whether the condition requires special treatment.

Regular Follow-up Visits

After the doctor has explained the nature of the disease to the patient and discussed the treatment plan with him he will ask him to come for regular periodic check-ups. At first, until the pressure is brought down to the level appropriate to his age or as close to it as possible, he will probably ask to see him more frequently, particularly since the lowering of the pressure is a gradual process (see p. 79) requiring constant checking. These frequent visits also afford the patient the opportunity to ask the doctor all the questions.

The actual blood pressure measurement is only one aspect of these visits. Your blood pressure, whether

Pressure can   treated or not, can vary, depending on the time of day, the
vary   weather, and any number of physical and psychological conditions (see p. 36). So it does not say very much about either the success or failure of the therapy if on different days the systolic pressure varies from 20 to 40 mm Hg and the diastolic pressure from 10 to 20 mm. What matters is whether the elevated pressure is the exception or the rule. Therefore the doctor at first will want to take as many readings as possible to help him to understand his patient's

88

condition. However, the kind of close control, so desirable especially in the case of severe hypertension, is not always possible.

In recent years an increasing number of patients have been taught to check their blood pressure themselves. Initially doctors had great misgivings about this approach, but the results have generally been so encouraging that more and more patients are being instructed in it. The fear that patients may develop a control neurosis have proved groundless. The danger is no greater than with diabetics who check themselves. The home measuring has proved highly effective with patients suffering from severe and particularly malignant hypertension and with patients who had trouble bringing their pressure down to satisfactory levels. The spontaneous variation of the pressure which can show up in the comparatively infrequent checks by the doctor can give a distorted picture whereas regular home measurement can give a far more accurate picture and assist the doctor in developing a better, less hazardous drug program. There is also a hidden psychological advantage. By becoming involved personally the patient turns from a passive treatment object into an active assistant of the doctor. Ask your doctor whether home measurement would be advisable for you (see p. 108).

Measuring pressure at home

Once the blood pressure has been brought down the patient does not have to see the doctor more often than every few months. On that occasion he will check your heart and circulation, other risk factors as well as lab reports that might detect undesirable side effects.

8. What the Patient Must Do

It's your life

It is *your* health and the quality and length of *your* life we are dealing with. And these depend largely on your attitude and your actions. Your doctor can work out a detailed treatment plan, he can try to keep you well informed and guide you with patience and understanding. But the rest is up to you. Therefore you should learn how to live with your high blood pressure.

How to Live with High Blood Pressure

Because high blood pressure is a chronic disease it must be treated forever. Many people have difficulty accepting this fact or its consequences. In talks with my patients I try to help them come to terms with this, to help them understand the nature of their disease and to get them to cooperate with me in fighting it.

• *It is important to learn to relax*, not live in constant fear about your blood pressure and an occasional higher

91

reading. On the other hand one can't bury one's head in the sand and pretend that there's nothing wrong.

• *Re-examine your values and goals.* Use the discovery of your hypertension to take stock of yourself. Have you been trying to do too much? Does your job get you down? Do you think that the work you're doing is meaningless? Do you feel overwhelmed by the demands being made on you? Are you trying too hard to make more money?

See what you're missing

Having thought about these and similar matters you may find that you have been missing out on a lot of beautiful things that life has to offer. And you may also find that it is foolish to continue chasing after things that may not be all that important after all.

• *Practice self-discipline and live sensibly:* the fight against high blood pressure does not involve extraordinary measures. All you are asked to do is to take your medication regularly and probably make some changes in your eating and living habits. Some people have a problem about following the rules laid down. Self-control and self-discipline are needed, particularly if you are asked to give up something like a favorite dish or cigarettes. Most doctors realize, often on the basis of personal experience, that what they ask of their patients is not always easy. But that does not relieve them of the responsibility to convince their patients of the need for adherence to their orders.

Routine

The key to successful treatment

Routine is the key to successful treatment, and self-discipline is the key to routine. Here are some of the things you must do routinely:
• Take medication
• Stick to your diet
• Alternate work with rest and play

92

- Get enough sleep
- Exercise
- Go for checkups and have your blood pressure taken (or take it yourself)

Prevent serious disease

I know of only few cases where people could not adjust to the change in their lives. The thing you should keep in mind is that you can prevent your high blood pressure from turning into a serious disease.

Making Adjustments

I am often asked by patients what effect their sickness will have on their job or profession, what they can eat, whether they can engage in sports, what the treatment is like, what they are allowed to do on their vacations, whether they can drink alcohol or coffee or tea.

In the following sections I will try to answer these and related questions.

Your Job or Profession

Most people derive satisfaction from their work. It is a source of self-affirmation and lends meaning to their lives. But if they happen to suffer from high blood pressure they must arrange their work schedule so as to eliminate too much pressure and long, irregular hours. A long work day

Long work day problematical

with only a short lunch break becomes more problematical for the person with high blood pressure the older he gets, and the severity of his hypertension is directly related to the degree of difficulty and responsibility of his job. Coffee, nicotine or possibly even stronger stimulants are not the answer to afternoon fatigue, especially not if you have high blood pressure. Instead, try to get enough rest during your lunch break. Give yourself a chance to unwind and your blood pressure a chance to go down. If you do this you will come back in the afternoon relaxed and rested. Try to arrange your work schedule so that you can get this noonday rest.

In setting up your work schedule try to follow these rules:

• Avoid all extraneous stress and overexertion
• Avoid long hours, night work, or shift work
• Try to keep a regular schedule
• Lunch periods of at least 1 hour with short naps if possible

Ask your plant doctor for advice. In some rare instances a change of jobs may even be indicated. Hypertensives should avoid strenuous physical labor, especially if it involves lifting and carrying heavy loads, as well as jobs in which the possible side effects of their medication could affect their own safety and that of others, for example: truck drivers, airplane pilots, crane operators, construction workers, etc. If you have high blood pressure and are working in one of these fields try to get advice on retraining for another job or profession.

How to Spend Your Leisure Time

If you suffer from hypertension try to spend your leisure in ways that benefit your health. Of course you should be doing things you enjoy and that meet your needs. If you spend your work day sitting behind a desk you should try to do something physical in your free time, and if your work involves physical labor you should rest. But

whatever your job, try to make your leisure time activities serve your health needs. You might consider outdoor activities like walking, bicycling, fishing, outdoor games, gardening, or indoor hobbies like photography, film-making, painting, collecting, carpentry, raising flowers or animals, reading, listening to music or playing an instrument, taking courses, watching TV, going to the theater.

Moderate Physical Exercise Is a Must

Open air exercise

Daily physical exercise in the open air is essential. Ten minutes of exercising in front of an open window and a short walk in the evening are a minimum requirement. If you have not done any exercise for a long time start out slowly and gradually increase the time and degree. An exercise bicycle is another good way of working out; begin slowly and gradually increase. Once you have begun doing daily exercises you won't want to do without it. After only a short time you will notice the difference in your energy.

If you have a favorite sport or sports you will want to know whether you can go on doing it, or if you haven't been involved in any particular sport you may decide to take one up. Whichever it is, don't do anything without first talking to your doctor.

Recommended Sports

Light exercise recommended

Generally speaking all types of light exercise are recommended. If you love the outdoors you can take walking, bicycle or canoe trips or go rowing. Whether walking or bicycling or canoeing, start slowly and gradually build up to longer distances. Cross-country skiing is another ideal sport. It is easy to learn, involves almost every muscle, and because of its even rhythm is especially relaxing.

If you like ball games choose one that is relaxing rather

than competitive. Tennis depends on your attitude toward it, whether you play for fun or whether you go all out and play to the point of complete exhaustion. The same holds true for downhill skiing.

Swimming Swimming is another ideal activity. However, and this is important, never swim in water whose temperature is much below 68°F, and never swim if nobody else is around, particularly if you are on strong drugs. Immediate assistance must be available should you suffer a dizzy spell or faint. Thermal baths in water temperature above 80°F are permitted only if your heart is okay. If you are a good swimmer and enjoy the sport you probably won't get short-winded. If you do, swimming is not for you. Diving is definitely out.

If you find that walking isn't enough exercise for you you can work your way up to jogging. The best way to begin is to alternate ordinary walking, about 20 to 30 steps, with 20 to 30 steps of jogging. Begin with short distances and work up to longer ones. Never force the tempo.

Knowing When to Stop

Hypertensives must know when to stop even if they feel no strain while actively exercising. The limit for the patient with a well-regulated blood pressure is reached
Pulse rate when his pulse rate per minute is 180 minus his age. In
sets limit other words, if you are sixty, your pulse rate during exercise should not exceed 120 per minute. In case of coronary damage the stress limit may be somewhat lower. Have your doctor determine what it is. With limited cardiac capacity the ordinary pulse rate may be higher to begin with and go up precipitously with slight exertion. In that case your doctor may limit the physical activities.

96

Non-advisable Physical Exercises and Sports

Exercises demanding great sudden exertion or sustained effort as well as all athletic competitions are definitely out. This includes all sports involving pressure breathing that raises the blood pressure: boxing, sprinting, diving, discus and hammerthrow, push-ups, etc.

Vacations

Make your vacation serve your health needs by planning it carefully and in detail. Doctors are frequently asked how often should vacations be taken and for how long.

Switch off
It is important for people with high blood pressure to "switch off," to get away from their job with its attendant worries and problems. So if at all possible take two annual vacations of 1-2 weeks each.

When is the best time for a vacation? Avoid the summer crowds and hot months. That will not give you the needed rest. Spring and fall are far better times.

Where to go? The shorter and less strenuous the trip you take, the more remote and restful the area, the greater your chances of rest and relaxation. Wooded rolling hills or mountain foothills are ideal spots, but the seashore in mild climates is also recommended. Stay away from the tropics, however.

Avoid the tropics

Mountains. Elevations of between 1,300 and 2,600 feet are fine, although people with mild hypertension can tolerate heights of up to 5,000 feet. But if you have severe hypertension and congestive heart failure, elevations of more than 4,000 feet are definitely hazardous. And everyone with high blood pressure should avoid too rapid changes in altitudes, such as going up a mountain in a cable car.

97

Car travel. If at all possible leave your car at home, particularly if you are planning a long trip. One day behind the wheel is more strenuous than a full day's work. And without a car you will get more rest once you have arrived at your destination. For short trips try renting a bicycle. If you feel you absolutely must take a car, make frequent rest stops and if possible avoid driving on crowded highways.

Leave the car home

Flying. On short flights there are no great changes in cabin pressure and most patients can take such trips without running any risk. On long trips flying at altitudes of between 33,000 and 40,000 feet (equivalent to land altitudes of 6,500-8,000 feet) people with a controlled pressure generally fare quite well, probably because they are resting. But the rapid pressure changes in take-off and landing can cause serious problems. It therefore seems advisable that persons suffering from malignant hypertension (see p. 49), or persons whose pressure has not been controlled, who have cerebrovascular problems, angina pectoris, arrhythmias, coronary insufficiency, or are recovering from a recent heart attack, should not fly, or certainly not without first consulting their doctor. While flying avoid foods likely to produce gaseous distension ("gas"), carbonated beverages, and adjust your medication schedule to changes in the time zones.

Short flights no risk

Spas. European spas with mineral water cures should be avoided because of the high sodium content of most such waters. At any rate consult your doctor before taking any "cure".

Sunbathing and saunas. Overexposure to sun and heat are not advisable, especially if you are taking strong antihypertensive drugs. That means stay away from southern beaches. Moderate sunbathing in temperate climates and moderate physical activity are permitted. The heat of a sauna bath puts no greater strain on the heart and circulation than do swimming and jogging, but don't follow this by an ice-cold shower or plunge into an icy pool. This can drive your blood pressure up to dangerously high

Avoid overexposure

levels. Cool off before taking a cool shower. People with moderately high blood pressure generally have no trouble with saunas, but a long-range effect on the blood pressure is lacking. The decision in individual cases must be left to the doctor. Persons with very high or poorly controlled blood pressure or persons suffering from congestive heart failure or angina pectoris should stay away from saunas.

eep to your diet

Diet and medication. Don't deviate from your diet and don't stop taking your drugs while on vacation, even though your blood pressure may go down when you are relaxed. If you take your own blood pressure consult your doctor whether you can reduce the drug dosage when and if your pressure goes down. If you go to a foreign country be sure to take an adequate supply of your medication; it may not be available in the place you are visiting.

Coping with Stress in Daily Life

ome stress navoidable

There is no life without stress. Nervous and psychological stress is an unavoidable part of daily living. It is pointless and unrealistic to tell somebody to avoid stress and not get excited. How can one reduce stress? Logically and psychologically there are only two ways:
• By avoiding stress-producing conditions (see p. 22-23).
• By controlling one's reactions to known stress-producing factors.

How can these suggestions be translated into reality? Some stress-producing situations are avoidable without affecting any major aspect of our personal or professional lives, for example, avoidance of driving in rush-hour traffic, unnecessary family and job conflicts, overtime work or honorary posts, violent political arguments, exhausting meetings, and many similar daily activities that are not absolutely essential.

Yet all too frequently we are confronted by stressful situations that cannot be either avoided or changed. In

99

such a case the only thing we can do is to moderate our reaction to the situation, to get rid of the irritation as quickly as possible. Letting off steam rather than swallowing one's annoyance whether it involves a co-worker or friend or close relative, sometimes helps. Many people find release in physical exercise. In the case of long-standing career or personal problems you must develop a technique for coping with the stress. There are various ways of adjusting to the situation. Which one you choose, preferably with the help of an understanding counselor, depends on the nature of the problem and on your personality. The possibilities range from medication to relaxation techniques like yoga and meditation to psychotherapy.

Sleep

In conclusion I want to mention a simple and proven method of overcoming stress: restful sleep. Lack of sleep can make you stress-prone, and stress in turn keeps you from falling asleep. How does one break through this vicious circle and achieve the relaxation that makes sleep possible? Here are some tips that may help to overcome sleeping problems: physical exercise before going to bed, light reading while sipping a glass of wine or light beer before turning off the light. And if sleep still eludes you, try some relaxation techniques.

Sleeping pills

Sleeping pills, particularly in conjunction with alcohol, should be avoided. They can be addictive and do nothing to get to the cause of the problem. Occasionally lying awake is not such a bad thing. It gives you the chance to review your day and think how to cope with stress-producing problems.

Losing Weight by Eating Sensibly

Recently a patient of mine walked into my office and at first I simply couldn't recognize him. When I had last seen him a year earlier he was 50 lbs. overweight, his urine showed traces of sugar, his blood pressure was up to 220/130, and he could not understand why, despite the medication (which he took sporadically), his blood pressure refused to go down. I tried to tell him that obesity and hypertension was a particularly dangerous combination and that if he went on a diet his blood pressure was sure to go down. He promised to follow the diet I recommended, but I must admit that I was skeptical. So I was surprised when I saw him again. His weight was down to normal, as was his blood sugar; his blood pressure was 145/85 without the benefit of drugs and he had taken up tennis again. He proved what doctors know only too well: that in many cases blood pressure can be reduced or even brought down to normal levels if the patient would lose weight.

Dangerous combination

Obesity and blood pressure often go hand in hand, but few people want to face up to this or accept the fact that they have to lose weight. How often do doctors have to listen to patients who tell them that they have to eat a lot to be able to work.

The body uses up calories very sparingly, as the following table indicates. The figures given are the body's expenditure of calories per 30 minutes of the listed activity:

How body uses up calories

Activity	Calories
Driving	30
Walking (2 mi. per hour)	51
Polishing shoes	63
Light gymnastics	70
Bicycling with no crosswind (6¼ mi. per hour)	84
Painting walls	85
Running a vacuum cleaner	88
Cleaning windows	99
Lifting stones	108
Chopping soft wood	112

Sawing wood	154
Playing soccer	232
Long-distance running	
(6 mi. per hour)	340
Cross-country skiing	
(5 mi. per hour)	390

Men twenty-five years of age doing light physical work use up about 2,500 calories per day; women that same age doing light physical work use up an average of 2,100 calories daily. To arrive at your calorie expenditure deduct 100 calories for every fifteen additional years.

Heavy bones?

How often have you heard somebody say *"I have heavy bones."* The fact of the matter is all of us have bones and that they weigh between 18 and 22 pounds. *"My parents also had a large frame,"* or *"It's my glands"* are also favorite excuses. If you are overweight your body is getting more food than it can use up. True, some people burn up more calories than others doing the same amount of work, but if an entire family has a "large frame" it simply means that all of them eat improperly and have done so since childhood. There are rare cases where obesity is caused by a glandular disorder, but don't be your own diagnostician. Let the doctor determine the cause of your weight problem.

Weight and nerves

Many people feel that nerves should be "cushioned" in fat. They equate overeating with feeling relaxed, with escape from tension and worries. But overeating is the wrong type of relaxation. There are numerous ways of relaxing, from exercise to meditation.

Throw out those tired old alibis, get rid of your old-fashioned ideas of beauty and your old eating habits. Let me appeal to your vanity—thin is more beautiful than fat—and keep in mind that rich sauces, high-fat cheeses, cakes and sweets can shorten your life. Overweight is a health hazard for people with high blood pressure.

• Excess weight increases an already elevated blood pressure level

102

- Excess weight burdens your heart
- Excess weight increases the chances of acquiring additional risk factors like diabetes and metabolic disorders, e.g., hypercholesterolemia, and gout

What this adds up to is that the hypertensive patient must try to bring down his weight to normal, or better still, to ideal levels:

Ideal weight

- Ideal weight for women: normal weight minus 15%
- Ideal weight for men: normal weight minus 10%

There are two things you must do, and do consistently, if you are to achieve this goal:

To avoid putting on weight or to lose excess weight, *be calorie-conscious in eating.*

Eat a low-salt diet to support the effectiveness of your antihypertensive medication.

Be calorie-conscious

A few basic hints

This is not a book on how to lose weight, and so it will give you only a few basic hints on sensible eating and weight control as they relate to the problem of hypertension. The most important factor in a weight control program is a quantitative and qualitative change in your diet. What does that mean? First of all, that you give your body fewer calories than it uses up. You must decrease the calories in your diet while retaining its nutritional value.

Before you can do this you must find out the caloric value of the foods you eat and their vitamin and mineral content. I tell my overweight patients to write down everything they eat every day, and then translate the daily total into calories. By everything I mean exactly that: all the snacks and soft drinks, as well as the regular meals.

My reason for asking them to do so are (1) they learn about the caloric and nutritional value of the foods they eat, and (2) by adding up their total daily calories they find to their astonishment that they eat more than their body can use up.

103

A normal balanced diet should be composed of 12-15% proteins, 30-35% fats, 50-60% carbohydrates. In a weight-reducing diet you can cut down on both the fats and the carbohydrates, but try to keep the protein content high and get your carbohydrates mainly from whole-grain breads and cereals, unpolished rice, vegetables, potatoes, and fresh fruit.

A balanced diet

In eating refined sugar you are eating "empty" calories, that is, calories that do not supply the body with essential nutrients. Substitute artificial sweeteners that contain neither calories nor carbohydrates for refined sugar.

Watch out for hidden fats in your diet: 3½ oz. of bologna contains 1.8 oz. fat, 3½ oz. whipped cream 1 oz., and 3½ oz. of herring filets .8 oz. Use polyunsaturated fats (e.g., safflower, sunflower, soya bean oil, margarine) instead of butter.

Eat more often

We know from experience that people can lose weight more easily if they eat more often, that is to say, if they spread out their total daily calories over five or six smaller meals instead of the traditional three. In rearranging your meal schedule make these in-between meals high in proteins and low in carbohydrates.

To spare you the trouble of constant calorie-counting, I suggest that you set yourself a goal of the weight you want to lose in a week. Then try to figure out by how many calories you must reduce your diet to reach the goal without feeling too weak. Then work out your own reducing plan and stick to it until you have come down to your normal, or your ideal weight.

Some suggestions

Here are some suggestions that will help you acquire better eating habits: set definite meal times and don't eat in-between; eat slowly; don't watch TV or read while eating; serve smaller portions on smaller plates; interrupt your meal with telephone conversations, etc.; throw away all leftovers when finished eating; don't leave any food and/or drinks standing around within easy reach.

Changing old habits is difficult; don't get discouraged. Once you have become calorie-conscious you will be able

104

to stop counting the calories of every bite you eat. Also, don't be discouraged if at first you don't lose as much weight as you expect even though you follow your diet. The reason you may not is the change in your metabolism

Be patient and water and hormonal balance. Be patient, you are sure to lose weight, and with it bring down your blood pressure.

Then, proud and pleased with yourself about having come down to your normal or ideal weight, stick to your new, sensible diet (see p. 104). Make sure that you continue to eat balanced meals and that you get enough minerals and vitamins. And remember: with every pound you gain back you increase the risk that your blood pressure will go up again.

If you should relapse and your scale tells you that you have regained some of the weight you had lost, then one day a week eat only raw foods: dry whole grain cereals, salads without oily dressings, fresh fruit.

To lose weight rapidly, limit your diet to these totals given by Dr. S. Heyden in his book *Risk Factors of Ischemic Heart Disease* (however, do this on your vacation, not when you're working):

Medical recommendations for weight reduction

1. Replacement of sodium by herbs and spices

2. Restriction of carbohydrates to 60 g per day (= 240 calories)

3. Normal protein ingestion of 60 g (= 240 calories)

4. Limitation of fat intake to 25 g (= 225 calories)

5. One fasting day per week. Only non-caloric liquids are permitted

105

6. Keeping a diary of food intake

7. Daily weight recording in the morning

8. 150 calories for breakfast
   150 calories for lunch
   400 calories for dinner

9. The sodium restriction may be lifted after 8-10
   weeks for persons with normal blood pressure
   levels.

Low-salt diet

Rule of thumb

Today we no longer prescribe an almost salt-free (.035 oz. per day), difficult to adhere to diet. Rather, we recommend a slight reduction in salt consumption ($^1/_{10}$-$^1/_5$ oz.). We prescribe diuretics to help the kidneys excrete the excess sodium. Follow this rule of thumb: no salt in the kitchen, no salt at the table. That means, never add salt to your food. In addition, all highly salted foods such as ham, pickled meats, sausages, marinated foods, salted cheeses and butter, prepared spicy sauces are taboo. It does not mean that meals have to be bland. There are many herbs that can lend flavor and interest to your meals. Once you develop a taste for them you will no longer miss the salt. The advantage of this diet is that it can be followed easily whether at home or eating out and protects the hypertensive patient from eating more salt than diuretics can help him excrete.

Special diets

These may be indicated if, even with normal weight, such metabolic disorders as diabetes, hypercholesterolemia, or hyperuricemia persist.

What You Can—and Cannot—Eat and Drink

Coffee and tea

To begin with: almost none of your favorite beverages if taken in moderation are forbidden. **Coffee and tea** in moderate quantities pose no problems for most people. As a matter of fact their stimulating properties can counteract the fatigue brought on by some of the medications. Some people, however, do experience unpleasant side effects such as overstimulation, palpitations, and/or a rise in blood pressure. They should stay away from these beverages. Too much and very strong tea and coffee are undoubtedly harmful for hypertensives if they are used to fight normal fatigue and as a substitute for rest.

Alcohol

Alcoholic beverages in moderation are permitted in the absence of other health problems such as liver disease. After a tough day at work a glass of wine or beer can be very relaxing. But you should know that alcohol can also intensify the fatigue factor of some drugs (see p. 87) to the point that driving becomes a hazard (see p. 113). Because alcohol is highly caloric and stimulates the appetite it should be kept to a minimum, and omitted altogether while on a reducing diet. If you have a weight problem, drink low-calorie beverages and avoid hard liquor. A bottle of champagne may not affect your blood pressure but it will add 1,000 calories to your diet.

Smoking

Smoking in every form and case is harmful. Cigarettes are a real risk factor, although cigars and pipes are also not advisable. Although it is true that less nicotine is absorbed through the mucous membranes than through inhalation into the lungs, pipe and cigar smokers will be tempted to inhale. As a rule it is easier to stop smoking altogether than to cut down to one or two cigarettes a day or to switch from cigarettes to cigars or a pipe. The only thing that works, and works immediately, is stopping altogether.

Drug Therapy

*Take your
medication*

This is merely a brief reminder of the importance of taking the medication prescribed to you by your doctor, and sticking to it. Here is what can happen if you ignore it or forget it:

• A sudden interruption of antihypertensive drugs can trigger a dangerous rise in pressure.

• Failure to take medication regularly can desensitize your body to antihypertensive drugs.

• Changing medication or its dosage without your doctor's permission can be dangerous and make you a hazard in traffic or at your job.

How to Take Your Own Blood Pressure

The method of taking blood pressure, whether by the doctor or the patient, has not changed since its invention by Dr. Riva Rocci (RR) and Dr. Korotkoff at the beginning of this century. It is still the most reliable and simplest procedure for determining the degree of arterial blood pressure.

This is how it works: an inflatable cuff connected to a pressure gauge (manometer) is wrapped around the arm above the elbow. By pumping air into the cuff with a rubber bulb the air pressure at a given point will stop the blood flow through the main artery in the arm. This pressure is registered on the manometer. To make certain that the arterial circulation has in fact been cut off, the pressure is increased by another 10-20 mm Hg. A stethoscope placed against the crook of the elbow picks up the sound of the pulse as the air pressure is released. As soon as the air pressure drops below the systolic pressure—i.e., the "peak pressure" of the pulse (see p.

*Systolic
pressure*

108

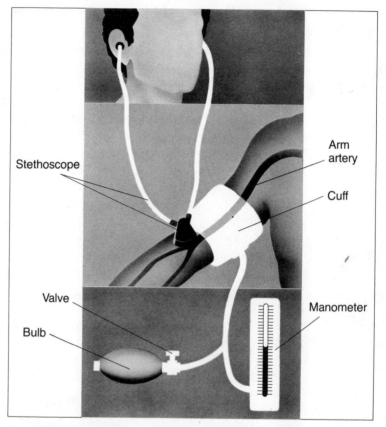

Reading the systolic and diastolic blood pressure values. The systolic blood pressure is indicated on the manometer scale when, after pressure has been lowered in the cuff, the artery's pulse beat again becomes audible in the bend of the elbow. The diastolic blood pressure is indicated on the manometer scale when the artery's pulse beats vanish after further lowering of pressure.

41)—thudding sounds produced by the blood being pushed through the previously constricted artery with every heart beat are heard in the stethoscope. As the air pressure continues to be eased, rhythmic sounds disappear at the very moment that the air pressure falls below the diastolic pressure—i.e., when the spasmodic pulsation disappears even at the point of its lowest pressure. The manometer

Diastolic pressure

reading at this point of cessation gives the diastolic pressure.

Spotting errors in technique

A patient taking his own blood pressure must learn to spot the possible errors in his technique and how to get an accurate reading that will be of use to his doctor.

• He should take his blood pressure twice a day at identical times on the same arm (either right or left) while lying down (sitting) and standing.

• The arm must be free and unconstricted (e.g., no rolled-up shirt sleeve). The elbow should be held exactly at the same level as the heart.

• The cuff must be deflated and the stethoscope placed against the artery that runs along a line inside the upper arm to the center of the crook of the elbow.

• Because many people for some unknown reason have a silent zone—the so-called auscultory gap—between the systolic and diastolic pressure in which no pulse can be picked up by the stethoscope, the air pressure in the cuff must be pumped up to a point above the systolic pressure.

• The patient should keep a record of the daily pressure readings together with the drugs taken as well as his activities during the day.

• Sphygmomanometers (apparatus used to measure blood pressure) for home use should be standard, officially approved instruments, and be checked for accuracy at least once every two years.

Remember, home measurements do not mean home treatment. Changing medication and dosage, whether upward or downward, can only be done with your doctor's permission.

Patients and Their Spouses

Whether or not high blood pressure will create new and serious problems in a marriage depends both on the people involved and on the seriousness of the disease. The adjustments required of a patient with only a slightly elevated pressure are minor and do not really change the

110

rhythm of everyday life, but serious hypertension, perhaps complicated by heart disease or stroke can cause profound changes in personal relationships.

You, whether you are the patient or the partner, can make things either easier or more difficult. Sometimes serious hypertension compels the stricken partner or both to forgo some of their old favorite activities such as seashore vacations, long car trips, mountain climbing, downhill skiing, or party-going. If this is felt as a major deprivation a formerly good marriage can suffer. This writer has found that almost all couples who were willing to face up to their problems and seek a constructive, mutually satisfactory solution were able to find one. As a matter of fact the disease may even strengthen and deepen their feelings and mutual concern.

You can make things easier

The spouse can help through patience, understanding and support, by going along with some of the recommended changes in diet, exercise, smoking, etc. Occasionally the spouse must take the responsibility of seeing that the patient follows doctor's order, without constant reminders and nagging. However, it would be a serious mistake to put the entire burden and responsibility for following the recommended diet, rest, exercise, and medication on the shoulders of the spouse. Of course the patient must contribute to a satisfactory adjustment to changes in their lives by following the recommended treatment, enjoying the things that are allowed, avoiding moodiness, impatience, and irritability. The leisure time activity of the hypertensive woman, whether working and/or running a household, poses a special problem. She should be given a chance for a rest in the middle of the day and regular time off essential to relaxation and rest.

Patience, under- standing, support

People who have no problems in their marriage may find this advice, which applies to all chronic diseases, both trite and superfluous. But others are grateful if their doctor discusses these possible points of friction. These lines were meant for them.

111

9. Things You Must Also Know

Hypertension and Driving

Drugs and driving

Some antihypertensive drugs, particularly reserpine and clonidine (see p. 87) especially if taken in high dose or if the pressure has been brought down too abruptly, can slow down reactions and affect driving ability. That, however, is not an argument for letting hypertension go untreated, because the untreated patient may also be a driving risk. The untreated hypertensive faces other hazards which can be triggered by strain while driving: coronary patients can have attacks of angina pectoris (see p. 56), patients with cerebrovascular problems can suffer dizziness and fainting spells or be disabled by a sudden retinal hemorrhage. Also, kidney failure, cluster headaches, the sensation of things dancing before one's eyes, and above all, diminished reactions, can seriously impair the driving ability of hypertensives.

Persons receiving medication can experience fatigue, dimished reactions or acute attacks of weakness especially in conjunction with even small quantities of tranquilizers or alcohol, or if a high pressure was brought down too rapidly and abruptly rather than slowly and gradually.

If the blood pressure was taken with the patient sitting or lying down but not when standing, a possible tendency toward a drop in blood pressure will not have been

113

detected. Hazardous "orthostatic" reactions can also crop up after someone has been sitting for a long time, particularly older persons, either spontaneously or in the case of methyldopa and/or guanethidine treatment.

Caution is also advised in case of diuretic-induced potassium loss, leading to a decrease in the serum potassium level.

If you are taking drugs, particularly if yours is a serious case of hypertension, be sure to check with your doctor whether it is advisable for you to drive.

Rules for driving
If your doctor says it is, keep 8 rules in mind:

1. Don't take any pain killers, mood drugs, sleeping pills, or alcohol.
2. Don't change drugs or dosages on your own.
3. Take your blood pressure regularly and go for regular checkups.
4. Don't drive when starting out on or changing medication.
5. Avoid areas with low-oxygen levels (high altitudes, smoking in cars).
6. Avoid sudden physical exertion (changing tires, lifting heavy loads).
7. Don't drive long distances without frequent rest stops.
8. Stop driving immediately if you feel faint, tense, or if your concentration is slipping.

If you are under drug treatment for hypertension and drive remember that by ignoring this advice you can endanger not only yourself and your passengers but innocent bystanders as well.

High Blood Pressure— Contraception—Pregnancy

If you suffer from hypertension you should avoid oral

114

contraceptives because they may elevate the blood
pressure (see p. 46). Consult your gynecologist or a
contraceptive clinic for advice about alternative methods
of contraception. If you are not planning on any more
children or if the termination of a pregnancy is medically
indicated, you might consider sterilization as the most
reliable and safest method of contraception. This procedure does not affect the production of female hormones
nor the sex life. If you are planning to have children
consult your doctor about the advisability of a pregnancy.
Some types of hypertension can produce serious complications that could endanger the life of the mother and the
fetus. If a previous pregnancy has been complicated, or in
the case of malignant hypertension (see p. 49) or advanced
hypertension with impaired kidney function the pregnancy
may have to be terminated. A hypertensive woman who
finds that she has become pregnant should consult her
doctor promptly to determine whether she can carry her
child to term. If she does, she should have regular monthly
checkups in the early stage of her pregnancy and biweekly
checkups in the later stage. She should check both her
weight and blood pressure daily and keep a written record
(see p. 108). If her blood pressure is only slightly or
moderately elevated her doctor may take her off
medication during the first four or five months, even
though the medication is harmless. During this period he
may want to rely on the antihypertensive effects of a
strictly low-salt diet.

Oral contra-
eptives can
elevate
pressure

The "Hypertensive Patient's I.D."

Like diabetics or people taking anticoagulants, hypertensives should carry identifications that state the type and
dosage of the medication they are taking, their most recent
blood pressure reading, and the name and address of their
doctor. Ask your doctor to get you such a form.

The 12 Basic Rules for Hypertensives

Here in a nutshell are the most important rules you should follow and remember:

Important rules

1. Have your blood pressure checked regularly or take it yourself.
2. Cut down on salt.
3. Lose weight.
4. Take the drugs prescribed by your doctor.
5. Give up smoking.
6. Cut down on alcohol.
7. Exercise regularly.
8. Avoid pressure and stress.
9. Get enough sleep; learn to relax.
10. Let your doctor decide whether you are fit to drive.
11. Take a vacation of at least 1 to 2 weeks.
12. Exercise caution in altitudes of more than 5,000 ft., sudden changes of climate, and while flying.

10. The Future Outlook

Perhaps you will read this last chapter first. You may have found out only recently that your blood pressure is high and this may depress and frighten you. If so, this chapter should give you confidence and optimism.

You will have to accept the fact that high blood pressure is a chronic, and except for some rare, surgically curable forms, life-long disorder which cannot be ignored. But the treatment involved does not make impossible demands on you. You can go on living the way you have been with some changes to which you can adjust as quickly as to the need for medication. If you find these rules difficult remember that proper treatment can bring down your pressure and prevent dangerous heart and brain complications. Some cases of essential hypertension have even disappeared after blood pressure was normalized for an extended period, which calls into question the theory of incurability. The medical profession therefore justifiably

Justifiable optimism feels more optimistic than ever before. Of course, without the cooperation of the patient we doctors cannot succeed. Help your doctor by being an intelligent, cooperative partner. You both want the same thing: to treat your hypertension successfully and help you lead a normal, productive life.

Postcript for Doctors

Recent epidemiological studies prove beyond any doubt that the already low compliance with doctors' orders by patients with chronic diseases is particularly low among hypertensives. One of the reasons as we all know is the fact that hypertensives often feel well and energetic and do not experience their hypertension either as an impairment or as a threat. Like the obese patient the hypertensive's "cognitive dissonance" is supported by the absence of discomfort, and thus lacking overt symptoms, he is more likely to ignore medical advice. Another reason for the poor response of hypertensives to medical advice is the lack of information (substantially below the awareness of diabetics) about the nature, hazard, and necessity for treatment.

Only recently have efforts to raise public awareness been intensified. Yet at the same time studies have shown that more information can also have negative effects. For example, the recent augmentation of information about drugs and their possible side effects has made many people reluctant to take pills. The listing of the potential side effects on the labels has aroused widespread fears. The patient is told about the danger of a given treatment but nothing about the need for and success of the therapy.

Thus he is unable to weigh its potential risks against the great hazards of untreated hypertensive disease.

This makes it incumbent upon us not to let up on our efforts to counteract ignorance and misunderstanding with information and motivation. It has been my experience that people with chronic diseases, and hypertensives in particular, listen to their doctor only if the nature of their disease has been explained to them and they understand the need for cooperation and regular checkups. That is a time-consuming process, and even then misinformation can continue to flourish. A recent study showed that 70% of all patients have forgotten vitally important instructions five minutes after leaving the doctor's office.

That is why I have tried to emphasize the importance of the doctor-patient relationship. In addition, I am sure that even doctors who have spent a lifetime fighting this epidemiologically most widespread disease of our time cannot confine themselves simply to the purely medical and scientific area. I was therefore glad to be able to contribute this volume to the *Medical Adviser Series*. I knew before I began that it would not be easy to render medical information in terms understood by the layman. I have tried to give the patient objective information about high blood pressure without creating insecurity through medical half-education, and to motivate him psychologically to cooperate in his treatment without exaggerating the dangers.

If in your opinion I have not always succeeded in what I have set out to do, you can help me by suggesting revisions for future editions. Write to me which sections you feel could stand clarification and improvement. Send an annotated copy to the publisher who will gladly replace it with a new desk copy.